LAST
WRITES

WRITING LIVES
ETHNOGRAPHIC NARRATIVES

Series Editors:
Arthur P. Bochner and Carolyn Ellis
University of South Florida

Writing Lives: Ethnographic Narratives publishes narrative representations of qualitative research projects. The series editors seek manuscripts that blur the boundaries between humanities and social sciences. We encourage novel and evocative forms of expressing concrete lived experience, including autoethnographic, literary, poetic, artistic, visual, performative, critical, multivoiced, conversational, and coconstructed representations. We are interested in ethnographic narratives that depict local stories; employ literary modes of scene setting, dialogue, character development, and unfolding action; and include the author's critical reflections on the research and writing process, such as research ethics, alternative modes of inquiry and representation, reflexivity, and evocative storytelling. Proposals and manuscripts should be directed to abochner@cas.usf.edu.

Volumes in this series:

Erotic Mentoring: Women's Transformations in the University
    Janice Hocker Rushing

*Intimate Colonialism: Head, Heart, and Body
in West African Development Work*
    Laurie L. Charlés

Last Writes: A Daybook for a Dying Friend
    Laurel Richardson

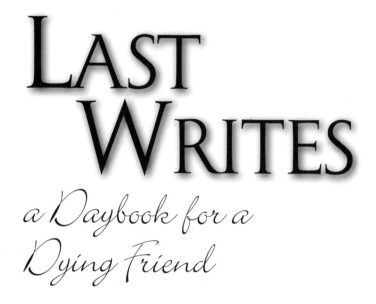

LAST WRITES

a Daybook for a Dying Friend

LAUREL RICHARDSON

Left Coast Press Inc.   Walnut Creek, California

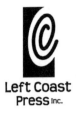

Left Coast Press Inc.

LEFT COAST PRESS, INC.
1630 North Main Street, #400
Walnut Creek, CA 94596
http://www.LCoastPress.com

ISBN 978-1-59874-186-5 hardcover
ISBN 978-1-59874-187-2 paperback

Library of Congress Cataloguing-in-Publication Data
Richardson, Laurel.
    Last writes : a daybook for a dying friend / Laurel Richardson.
        p. cm. — (Writing lives—ethnographic narratives)
    ISBN-13: 978-1-59874-186-5 (hardback : alk. paper)
    ISBN-13: 978-1-59874-187-2 (pbk. : alk. paper)
    1. Female friendship.   2. Richardson, Laurel—Diaries.   3. Kirschner, Betty Frankel.   4. Terminally ill—Biography.   I. Title.

BF575.F66R53 2007
177'.62—dc22   2007018703

Printed in the United States of America

♾™ The paper used in this publication meets the minimum requirements of American National Standard for Information Sciences—Permanence of Paper for Printed Library Materials, ANSI/NISO Z39.48–1992.

07 08 09 10 11 5 4 3 2 1

Original paintings on the cover, "Moon Rock" and the chapter openings, "White Nights," were provided by Ernest Lockridge.

Text design by Detta Penna
Copyediting by Sandra Craig

DEDICATED TO THE MEMORY

OF

BETTY FRANKEL KIRSCHNER

...number our days that we might gain a heart of wisdom. . . .

Psalm 90

He's not the finest character that ever lived but he's a
human being and a terrible thing is happening to him.
So attention must be paid.

Death of a Salesman, Arthur Miller

CONTENTS

About the Author

Laurel Richardson is Professor Emeritus of Sociology at The Ohio State University. She specializes in qualitative methodology, gender, the sociology of knowledge, and arts-based research. She has been honored with visiting lectureships in many countries, most recently in Denmark, Iceland, and Australia, where she was a Distinguished Fellow at the University of Melbourne.

Richardson has published more than one hundred articles, many of them demonstrating alternative writing formats. She has written definitive articles for various handbooks, including "Writing as Method of Inquiry," in the *Handbook of Qualitative Research* (edited by Denzin and Lincoln). She is the coeditor of *Feminist Frontiers* and author of six other books: *Dynamics of Sex and Gender*; *Gender and University Teaching: A Negotiated Difference* (Statham, Richardson, and Cook); *Writing Strategies: Reaching Diverse Audiences*; *The New Other Woman* (translated into seven languages); the Cooley-award-winning book *Fields of Play: Constructing an Academic Life* (Rutgers University Press); and *Travels with Ernest: Crossing the Literary/Sociological Divide* (AltaMira, coauthored with the novelist Ernest Lockridge). *Last Writes* is a continuation of her engagement with the theory, practice, and ethics of representation. She lives in Worthington, Ohio, with her husband, Ernest Lockridge, and their vociferous rescued red Abyssinian cat, Mimi.

PREFACE

Last Writes: A Daybook for a Dying Friend tells two interlocking stories. The first story is a friendship story, in which I tell of the last ten months of my best friend's life and of our thirty-five-year complex and sometimes difficult friendship, a deep friendship between two women. The second story is the story of the writing.

My original intention in keeping the Daybook was to help me endure my friend's terrible illness and death through an honest expression of my terribly mixed emotions—sadness, anger, disgust, fear—and by exploring more generally my attitudes toward death, dying, and friendship. A few months into the writing, I felt that my experiences were not unique. The death of friends is a major fact of life and, as baby boomers age, an increasingly prevalent fact. Because in two library searches I found no book about this, I thought the friendship story might be of value to others.

I also decided that the story of the writing, including ethical, writerly, and practical aspects, would be of interest to writers, researchers, and caretakers, both medical and nonmedical. And I thought the telling of the interlocking two stories through the format of the daybook would be of special value, interest, and support because grief work, like life work, is done day by day.

My hope is that this book will find its way into the hands of those who will discover in the interlinking stories ideas that ease their work, assuage their pain, and raise their awareness about death and dying in twenty-first century America.

Acknowledgments

Gratitude fills my heart and flows out in words of thanks:

To my husband, Ernest Lockridge, who has read every word in this manuscript, listened to it read aloud, cheered on my friendship with Betty, and supported me during the long months of her dying and the, aftermath of my grieving. He has generously provided his painting of "White Nights" for the chapter opening pages, and his painting of a full moon shining in Sedona for the cover.

To my memoir writing group—Beverly Davis, Nancy Lee, Diana Newman, Linda Royalty, Erica Scurr, Linda Thompson, and Deanne Witiak—who listened with great compassion and raised writerly questions with me.

To Maggie Kast, Susan Knox, and Carolyn Ellis, who read this manuscript and gave me thoughtful advice.

To Marilyn Falcouner, Ellyn Geller, Belinda Gore, Nancy Johnson, Patricia Lynch, Julie Miller, Merry Norris, Patricia Stuhr, Julie White, Mimi-the-cat, my Tuesday lunch group, and the postmodernist theory group, all of whom have helped me deal with my writing, pain, and loss, as did my wise, lovely, and nurturing sister, Jessica Phillips.

To Betty's family and friends, who helped her through her final days.

To the *Writing Lives: Narrative Ethnography Series* editors, Carolyn Ellis and Art Bochner, who have shared with me over the years, and now especially, their generous spirits, emotional presence, and intellectual gifts. Carolyn has in addition been my colleague, booster, and fellow beach-walker.

To the production crew, especially designer Detta Penna, copyeditor Sandra Craig, and cover designer Andrew Brozyna.

Last but far from least, to Mitch Allen, whose vision over the years, and now in creating Left Coast Press, Inc. has provided a meaningful space for work like mine.

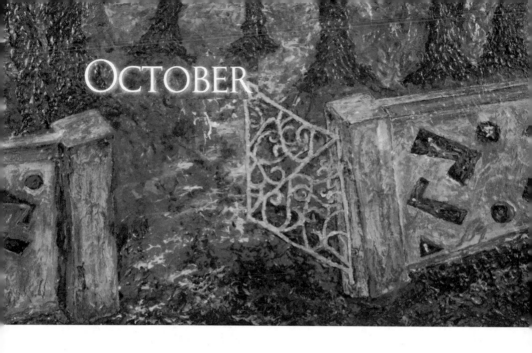

OCTOBER

Sunday, October 2

Last night I dreamt that my pearl necklace was holding on with but one thread.

Monday, October 3

A nurse calls and tells me that Betty is not doing well and has been admitted to the intensive care unit. On the hospital forms Betty has declared me her sister. We are not real sisters. We are best friends. We have been best friends for thirty-five years.

I drive the two hours from my home in Worthington, Ohio, to Robinson Memorial Hospital near Kent, Ohio. Betty is in intensive care. She looks like a wizened child, gray and small in a tussled hospital bed. I hold back my tears and hold her hand. Her chronic obstructive pulmonary disease (COPD)—emphysema and chronic bronchitis—has reached the perilous stage.

"She's bad," a nurse says. "Very bad. The attacks will only get more intense and closer together."

"She has two paths open to her," the pulmonologist says, "to be intubated, which she has refused, or to be made comfortable."

"I've been ready to pass over for the past six months," Betty says to me, once the nurse and doctor have left her room. "But I don't go. Why is it so much work?"

Betty taught sociology at Kent State University—Trumball Campus for thirty years, raised her daughter, Penny, worked in union and civil rights movements, and lived independently, keeping her dignity and sense of humor through years of increasingly ill health.

"Maybe because you've worked your whole life, you're working now too," I say. I think people often do their dying the way they do their living.

"It's not supposed to be this way," she says.

"How's it supposed to be, Betty?"

"You're supposed to get sick and just die."

But Betty's mother languished for years dying of stomach cancer. Her father drove his car into a light pole when he was eighty. It is his uncomplicated death that gave her money for a home-care assistant and a down payment on the house Penny and her husband, Mike, are building in rural Delaware. There'll be an attached apartment for Betty.

"The truth is I'm *not* ready to go," Betty says.

"I'm not ready either. . . ." *I don't know how I'll live my life without her.* "For you to go."

"There's still something left for me to do. Some ass to kick."

"Or maybe some slots to play."

"You bet."

Betty loves casino slots, betting on horses, betting on sports, playing the lottery. In this regard we differ. Games of chance bore me. I like duplicate bridge, a game Betty's never played.

After I check into my motel room, I open my Daybook. Writing is my primary way of handling stress, fear, and anxiety. As it is my habit to write every day, I write about my day, about Betty, about our friendship.

One of the most perfect days in my life I shared with Betty nearly thirty-five years ago. Both Betty and I were divorced at the time, her ex-husband was taking care of Penny, and my ex-husband was taking care of my preadolescent sons, Ben and Josh. Betty and I would have the day just for ourselves.

In the morning we went to a street fair and walked around the brightly colored tents set about the Worthington Village Green, turning my little town into a bedouin bazaar. In the afternoon we went to the Whetstone Park of Roses, where the heritage roses were in full bloom and, unlike the hybrids, smelling like roses. We sat at the lone picnic table, feasted on Katzinger's corned beef sandwiches on New York Jewish rye, and talked, without restraint, about the things that mattered to us. In the evening we went to Mershon Auditorium at The Ohio State University, where I taught sociology and Betty was one of my graduate students. We went to hear Vladimir Horowitz.

Our seats were foldaways set up on the stage. We could see Horowitz's breathing, feel his lightning intensity, totally immerse ourselves in the near-mystical experience—Horowitz and the concert grand seemingly one entity, no separation between the player and the played, and by extension no separation between the music and the listener. And what music! Clementi, Schumann, Scriabin, Chopin, Rachmaninoff. Mazurkas, ballads, sonatas.

At the end of the concert, silence prevailed throughout the auditorium, like the deep quiet before a storm—and then the storm, a thunderous crescendo, a stand-up ovation for minutes and more minutes. An encore, standing ovation, and then silence. Another encore, another standing ovation, and more sweet, sweet silence. The concertgoers milled about, nodding and smiling at each other but not talking, not normalizing or reducing the experience to ordinariness with after-concert banter. Perhaps a half hour later, people began filing out in silence, the way pilgrims do when they depart a sacred space.

Betty and I have been deeply bonded ever since we shared this perfect day.

Tuesday, October 4

Penny reaches me on my cell phone in Betty's hospital room. "Good news, Betty," I say. "Penny's crossed the bridge into Ohio. She'll be here in an hour."

"Then we've got some writing to do," Betty says. Her hand is swollen from steroids, bruised from IVs, and purple with vasilitis. She cannot hold a pen.

I take my spiral notebook and Bic pencil from my purse. "Tell me what you want me to write."

"Betty Frankel Kirschner died after being screwed around for five years by a variety of illnesses. Ms. Kirschner was the adoring mother—"

"Just a sec," I say. "I need to fix the lead."

"—of Penny Kirschner Smith and doting grandmother of Jack Smith. After graduating from Weequahic High School in Newark, New Jersey—that's where Phillip Roth went and—"

"Yah—but tell me about you, Betty."

"My older double-cousin Hettie Cohen married LeRoi Jones. I was a character in one of his plays."

"Do you want that in your obituary?" I ask.

"I don't think so." Betty looks dreamy. "Visits to them in Greenwich Village were some of the best times in my life. We went to jazz clubs, poetry readings, parties. . . . I learned about life. . . . I held their babies. . . . LeRoi abandoned Hettie and changed his name to Amiri Baraka . . ."

"So what about *you*?" My question breaks her reverie.

"Oh, okay. I . . . no, *she* taught at West Kinney High School in Newark for seven years. She completed her master's in sociology at the University of Alabama. She taught at Rutgers University and the University of Alabama at Tuscaloosa before she settled at Kent State University, where she taught for thirty years."

"A lifetime!"

"She took great pride in teaching working-class students, founding Sociologists for Women in Society, and organizing at the local, state, and national levels for the American Association of University Professors. She loved traveling and visiting her daughter, and was very blessed by her loyal, special friends, Laurel Richardson and Al Nelson."

"And?" I ask.

"That's it," she says.

"But what about your other friends and relatives?"

"No."

"How about, 'Betty Kirschner is sorely missed by her relatives and a host of friends?'"

"I guess . . . okay."

We make plans for a memorial service.

"At Bonnie's house?" I ask. Bonnie's house, an updated and enlarged farmhouse, with a three-tier deck and swimming pool, is situated on fourteen acres of grass, creek, and woods on a road outside of Kent. She had hosted the wedding reception for Penny and Mike. At the reception I mingled with Betty's friends from "The Union," the American Association of University Professors (AAUP). Their comments about Betty come back to me now: *courageous; feisty; New York edginess; passionate about social justice; romance fiction reader; casino devotee; music lover; good political advice giver; good eater; Trivial Pursuits maven.*

"Bonnie's house," Betty agrees.

The Kent people have known Betty in a different way than I have known her. Her public persona is political activist. She is an effective union organizer and negotiator. But the private Betty, the vulnerable Betty, has concealed her hand from them and shown it to me.

"Get the good caterer," she orders.

"Okay . . . Great Lakes Bakery," I say, recalling it from Penny's wedding.

"Have people speak about me," Betty says. "Memories, appreciations, laughter."

"Okay." We've talked about our memorial services often because we have totally different ideas about the open mike. It takes guts to want just anyone saying anything they want about you, behind your back, no less. Save me from that!

"Play music." She waves toward her bed stand, her purse.

I open the purse. Next to her half-smoked pack of Larks is an aged folded paper. I remove it.

Betty nods.

I unfold the paper. She has penciled—who knows when?—Schubert's Piano Quintet, "This Land Is Your Land," and "I Am Woman."

"Anything else?"

"Yeah, to be there," she says. "Just another party to which I am not invited."

"Your spirit will be there."

"You bet."

I wonder, What will I say at Betty's memorial service?
Betty and I were best friends. Are best friends.
We are sisters-by-choice.

Wednesday, October 5

When I came up to see Betty, I didn't realize I would be here for a few days. I need a clean shirt. I stop at the hospital gift store and get Betty some dark chocolate and myself a red T-shirt decorated with a faux-diamond dragon. A pair of slippers, the color of Sedona's red rocks, catches my eye, and I buy them too. In the lobby's restroom I don my new shirt and slippers.

"Ta-da! I'm dressed up in your honor," I tell Betty. She smiles at seeing me in a dragon shirt, her protective totem, but tears up when she sees my red slippers. She misses terribly the red rocks of Sedona.

"I'd like one of your kachinas," I say, surprised that I am actually asking for something I want.

"That makes me happy," she says. "I want you to have the Sunfaces." She's collected the kachinas on reservations, selecting each one from the artist who made it. Sunfaces are her favorites.

She looks thoughtful. She smiles and her face seems rounder, her complexion brighter, as if she's become a little Sunface herself. She says, "And I want you to have a long life, so I want you to have my pearls too."

Unlike my pearls, hers are large and have a clasp that allows you to wear them as a single or double strand. I've often admired them.

"I've brought you a present," I say, handing her a small book I made for her. Its spine is turquoise blue, and its cover paper looks like peacock feathers unfurled. On the end page I had calligraphed,

> *To my Best Friend,*
> *Betty*
> *For writing little thoughts & big ones*
> *Love,*
> *Laurel*

When I made the book and wrote those words, I didn't know that she'd have to think her thoughts, not write them.

She hugs the book to her heart tightly, as if doing so will magically transfer her thoughts to its pages or imbue it with her spirit.

Thursday, October 6

We discuss cremation and her burial at the foot of her father's grave in New Jersey.

"I'll turn off this overhead light," Nurse Beth says, coming in to check on the oxygen.

"No, you won't!" Betty looks squirrelly. "I want to be in the spotlight."

Friday, October 7

Penny's come and gone. "I'm glad you're here. You and Mom love each other," Penny said as we walked down the hospital corridor together. Her corn-colored ponytail, secured with a large heart-shaped barrette, swung freely over her XXL Red Dirt shirt. She held her package of Marlboros in one hand, her Bic lighter in the other.

Dr. Lillian Nash and two hospice workers came to Betty's room while I was soothing her, rubbing her hand. "You're doing all the right things," the hospice worker Jan says to me. Jan's been Betty's massage therapist for the past fifteen years. Jan makes house calls.

The hospice worker Carol gives Betty information on the program. "Going into hospice does not mean you have to die in six months—you can be renewed into the program indefinitely," Carol says. "And all your medical paraphernalia, medicines, and nursing visits would be 100 percent paid for."

Carol explains that Betty could be in the hospital hospice for three weeks or so and then go home or to a nursing home or back to the in-hospital hospice or whatever she chooses. She could change her mind in midstream. She would be totally in control. Hospice will give complete palliative care, neither preventing nor causing death.

"Will I be resuscitated?" Betty asks.

"No," Carol says, "in hospice, you won't be resuscitated, intubated, or brought to the ER."

"I've signed the papers transferring you to in-hospital hospice," Dr. Nash says. "We've done all we can. You're not going to get better."

I go into stillness, one of my ways of handling fear. I need to phone Penny. I hope I can tell her about her mom's prognosis without bursting into tears.

"I'll leave the hospice pamphlets here for you, Betty," Carol says.

"Would you like a little massage?" Jan asks. "It's on the house."

Saturday, October 8

On the drive back to Columbus, I feel a kind of peace taking me over. I've done everything I could with and for Betty. We've discussed leftover business. I apologized for not writing a letter in support of her try for promotion to full professor. Back then, some twenty-five years ago, I was totally vested in the norms and standards of academia. From my lofty vantage point at The Ohio State University, I thought her academic record did not justify promotion—even at a regional campus. Now, though, I would support her promotion. My greater understanding of the nature of regional campuses and my friendship with her would override my academic elitism.

As it turned out, she was promoted when she retired. Or so she told me. Why am I ruminating on this?

How remarkable that our friendship survived—survived the political, intellectual, and spiritual divergences that evolved between us over the years, and survived my getting married while she remained single. And survived her smoking!

When I get back home, my husband, Ernest, meets me eagerly. "I have a surprise for you," he says. In the living room he has propped up his first-ever paintings, three 36-by-48-inch acrylics, golden, yellow, and blue-hued knockoffs of Rothko—one of my favorite artists. "For you," he says, "to cheer you."

Sunday, October 9

When I call Betty this morning, she tells me the dream she had last night. "I was taking a long walk and looking for a secondhand store to put my things into," she whispers.

I like talking on the phone and I can easily settle into long conversations, often taking notes, writing down words. I was very nearsighted when I was young but wasn't fitted with glasses until I was a teenager. Listening became my primary way of apprehending the world. It still is. My career as an interviewer has been built upon my ability and desire to listen and remember what I have heard. I wait, wondering if Betty will say more about her dream. She doesn't.

"Listen to my dream," I say. "I am trying to find the eBay store that you've put your things into. I see it but I can't reach it. I don't have on the right shoes, it's getting dark, and the street has become a treacherous coastal path. I need to get home. There is snow and ice on the sidewalk now, so I walk in the middle of the street. An older black man walks beside me for a bit. 'I'm going home,' he says, and leaves. A young black man comes up beside me. 'You're alone,' he says. I pick up a handful of icy gravel and throw it at him."

"Once again, Laurel," Betty says, "we're sharing dreams. That's nice."

I've already interpreted my dream: *Betty will die in the wintertime. At first I will feel lost and scared, then I will have a guide, and no matter my fears, I will be able to take care of myself.*

Monday, October 10

I phone Dr. Nash, who informs me that Betty has decided not to go into hospice care. She wants to go to Regency Hospital for three weeks of rehabilitation therapy. Three weeks is the required minimum stay. The unit will continue to use the electric "pounders" on her lungs to loosen the solids that have formed. They will give her massages and physical therapy—moving her legs and trying to get her to walk to the bathroom. If she has another episode, she will be returned to Robinson and resuscitated.

"Hi, Betty," I say to her on the phone. "So you're going back to Regency." She'd been there twice recently.

"Yes," she whispers. "Talking to—what are they called—*hostile?*"

"Hospice, Betty. They're called *hospice.*"

"Talking to them now for the first time was helpful."

"Betty, you talked to them two or three times already. Carol spent over an hour with you two days ago."

"I don't remember," says Betty implacably. "I saw the hospice papers on my tray. I told them I want to go to Regency instead."

We talk some more.

"What are they called—*hostile*?" she asks again.

"*Hospice*!"

"Yes, hostile—they can't help me."

I have expended my energy on accepting her death, on believing she had accepted it too, getting hospice on board and offering her a solution that wouldn't make it "so hard" and "so much work." I had solved the problem to the best of my ability, and what has she turned around and done? Enrolled herself in a rehabilitation ward! Well, I am not going to go through all of this again. I am not going back to the hospital when she is brought back to the emergency room coughing and wheezing. I am not going to look at her in a respirator. I feel tricked, and ticked that she's rejected my help. I'm accepting her death. Why isn't she?

That night I dream that on my way somewhere else, I stop to drop off some things for Betty. Her barrel-chested baby is in the hospital with lung problems. The baby sits on an examining table, where I pet and soothe her. Betty sits nonchalantly some distance off.

"Can emphysema be inherited?" Betty asks the nurse.

"At times," the nurse answers.

"Bring me the bill, then."

When the nurse leaves, Betty says, "That's it. I'm going to sue this hospital!"

"What for?" I ask.

"Look how long it's taking to get the bill! *Once* I had to wait for a nurse!" Betty glares at me and says, "I don't want any more of your advice anymore either, Laurel!" Then she asks me to get her something and bring it back.

"Sorry," I say. "I'm on my way somewhere else."

Tuesday, October 11

"Look, this isn't about politics or movies or TV shows," Ernest says at breakfast, listing some of the things Betty and I habitually disagree about. "It's about dying. A person has every right to choose how they want to die. If Betty doesn't want to go into hospice, it's her choice."

Wednesday, October 12

I call Betty, who tells me she is restless and nervous, and that she's going home in four days. She's been in Regency for one whole day.

"No, Betty," I say. "You've committed yourself to three weeks."

"No one can tell me what I can or can't do!" she says. In my mind's eye, I see Betty's blue eyes glinting like diamonds.

When Betty was a kid and put to bed, she would keep herself awake by telling herself stories in which she was the princess, saved by a knight on a white horse. When she was a teenager, the knight became a virtuoso musician driving a white Jag. When a young adult, a lean, left-leaning politico saves her from a life of terminal boredom. "So you're bored in school," she had told her grandson, Jack, earlier this year. "Then tell yourself stories. You can do what you want in your stories. That's what I did. That's what I do."

Friday, October 14

"Ernest and I are off to Sedona tomorrow," I remind Betty on the phone. I've accepted the fact that her short-term memory is faulty. "We'll be gone two weeks plus."

"Bring me back some red sand from the other side of Cathedral Rock," she says. "You know where I mean."

Over the past fifteen years, Betty and I have often been in Sedona at the same time. She fell in love with a piece of for-sale land on Schoolhouse Road, on the north side of Cathedral Rock. She'd slowly walk about the plot of red earth, her head thrust forward like a turtle's, stepping around cacti, imagining the adobe house she would build. Of course there was no way she could ever afford that land—or the dream house—but I never disabused her of her fantasy. In her world, romance trumped reality.

Sunday, October 16

When Betty was twenty-three, she worked in a Jewish "Y" camp in Milford, Pennsylvania. Fifteen-year-old Ellyn was one of her campers. "Betty saved my life," Ellyn told me on the phone, "because she befriended and mentored me, insisting I go away to college, study psychology, and not teach in Newark." When Ellyn grew up, she opened a counseling practice in Princeton and gave Betty therapeutic advice. Ellyn and I have met twice and have bonded over our friendship with Betty. I can bad-mouth or praise Betty to Ellyn.

I get an e-mail from Ellyn at the Internet Café in Sedona:

Date: Sunday, October 16 10:40:58
From: ellyn336
To: richardson

Sunday a.m.

Yup. This is hard.

Someone just died in Betty's room last night. A young woman. Emphysema. Of course. Betty knew they weren't doing something correctly with the something. Still traumatic.

No complaints, however, with her care. Had sat up for 25 minutes.

Enjoy Sedona . . .

xo

Wednesday, October 19

"Happy *still* sixty-eight-year-old woman!" I am calling from Sedona. Betty is still in Regency. Her birthday is tomorrow. "What do you want for your birthday?" I ask.

"I have no wants left," she answers. "To go to a casino. To Sedona. And comfy shoes."

Thursday, October 20

"Happy sixty-ninth birthday! Did you have a good day?"

"I did." Betty sounds energized. "It was wonderful. Penny, Mike, and Jack all came from Delaware. Penny threw a party for me here in my room. David, Bonnie, Buzz, and Alfred came. They all gave me the same present—dark chocolate. I have enough dark chocolate to last me the rest of my life!"

Dark humor, huh, Betty? For more than twenty years, Betty had decided that she was allergic to chocolate and refused to eat it. Sometime this past year, though, she decided she wasn't allergic after all. Vintage Betty.

"Do you remember your sixtieth birthday here in Sedona?" I ask.

"How could I forget?" She's laughing.

On her sixtieth birthday, Betty arrived at the million-dollar, spanking new hacienda that Ernest and I were renting in Sedona (for a mere $2500 a month). She carried a Walgreen's plastic bag. Inside was Miss Clairol Permanent Color, Medium Warm Brown, specially formulated for fine, white hair like Betty's. My birthday present to her was to be my first (and last) dye job. I got brown dye all over the bathroom's pristine Southwestern accessories (Kokopelli light switches, coyote toilet paper holder, lizard-trimmed mirror, cacti toothbrush holders), and on Betty's Red Dirt T-shirt. We did girlish things, talked girly talk, acted silly. "Gotta pee?" she asked. "Yep," I said. When we're together for a bit, our need to pee gets synchronized. We were transported into an adolescence we hadn't had, either singly or together.

After the dye job, she thought she looked lovely, and her spirits soared. To me she looked older, her skin more sallow, her wrinkles more ridged.

Moroccan leather reclining chairs, black with mahogany arms, faced the largest and flattest television set I had ever seen. We sat down, reclined, and Betty hit the remote's power button. On came the news about the "wrongful death" civil suit against O. J. Simpson.

"O. J. didn't do it," Betty said.

"Are you serious?"

"Those L.A. cops framed him."

Betty's and my political divergence dates from that moment.

Now Betty says, "I'm glad you reached me at Regency. I'm going home in the morning. I didn't want you to worry if you called."

"Going home?"

"I'm having a hospital bed delivered."

I am silent.

"Penny and Mike will be there for my first night home."

I tell Ernest that Betty's going home.

"She'll be right back in the hospital," he says. "She'll smoke and that'll send her right back."

Friday, October 21

"Penny says you were up here for days, while I was in the hospital," Betty tells me on the phone.

"Well, I was there," I say.

"I don't remember."

"Well, I was there for five days."

"We wrote an obituary, didn't we?"

"Yes," I say. "And we planned the memorial service."

"My mind's protecting me," Betty says. "A panic attack. That's what happened."

Betty has a long history of panic attacks and agoraphobia. I don't know when, why, or how they began. Before I knew her, she had traveled widely throughout the United States and Europe. But about thirty years ago she developed a fear of flying—about the same time Erica Jong's book hit the best-seller list. I convinced Betty to just "try" by taking the short flight with me from Cleveland to Chicago for the sociology meetings. Throughout the flight she grasped the armrests and kept her eyes peeled on the cockpit door. Her breathing grew shallower. She was woozy when we left the plane. She took the train back to Cleveland. She did enroll in "fear-of-flying" classes but balked when the instructor expected her to enter a mock-up of a cockpit, so she could see the controls. "I don't like to be out of control," she said, when I asked her about her fear. She never flew again after our Chicago flight.

For the past thirty years, Betty's travels have been confined to the contiguous forty-eight states. Her travel has been complicated and increasingly dependent on the goodwill and services of others. To get her to Sedona, her friend Marty, who never sleeps, would drive her from Kent to Cleveland to catch the 4 a.m. train into Chicago. In the evening, she would take the overnight train from Chicago to Flagstaff, where the Little America van would pick her up at the station. The next day, the Enterprise Car company would bring her a car and she'd drive down Oak Creek Canyon to Sedona. Returning to Kent was equally complicated, time-consuming, and expensive. When she worked for the AAUP, they accommodated her fear and footed the extra travel and per diem expenses.

How admirable of Betty. Despite her agoraphobia, Betty did succeed in traveling. It took foresight, courage, and gumption more than I think I could have mustered.

Now we talk about her intensive-care-unit hospitalization.

"I've checked the web," Betty says. "I had an exacerbated lung attack. No explanation for it. Just have them and you either live or you die, but no one told me about that."

"Yes, they did. Twice," I say. "A real nurse and a real doctor. . . . So do you have your hospital bed?"

"Yeah. . . ."

"What's wrong?"

"It's a crummy Medicare bed. But it doesn't matter. I take a sleeping pill and then I wake up."

"Great that you can sleep."

"Penny tells me you were here for a few days. Thank you."

Saturday, October 22

"Hi, Betty, Ernest and I have had a great day! Drove up to Flagstaff, ate in a Thai restaurant, went to the Indian museum, to Snowbowl, rode on the ski lift to 12,500 feet where Navajo children were throwing snowballs, returned home, and got some great bread from Wildflower Bread Company." I stop for breath.

"I don't like their bread," she says. "It's pasty."

"But the company's only in Arizona and Utah."

"We have a Wildflower here," she insists.

"No you don't!"

"Whatever."

I feel like hanging up on her.

Sunday, October 23

I dreamt last night that I was up high on a ski lift and I tossed a baby down.

Tuesday, October 25

Today Ernest and I drove up Schnebly Hill and climbed on the Cow Pies, a dreadful name for one of the most beautiful spots in all of Sedona. The flattened red rocks look like humongous muffins about to rise, overlapped in a pan. Climbing on them I see before me all of Sedona, the Superstition Mountains, Mount Wilson, Cathedral Rock, Courthouse Butte. This is a place Betty and I used to visit. We'd sit here among the medicine wheels and dolmans, each in our own meditative space, welcoming the sacred, both wordlessly knowing somehow when it was time to move on. I call Betty to tell her.

"Wonderful. It makes me happy to know you are there," she says. Her breath is coming very hard, but I can hear Vivaldi in the background. Over the years, when she was not watching television, classical music filled the rooms, as it did when she was a child and her mother gave piano lessons.

"How's the smoking going?" I ask. Betty has been a die-hard smoker since she was thirteen. Even after she knew she had emphysema, she kept on smoking. I'm concerned, but it is ornery of me to ask because Betty's smoking has joined our pantheon of verboten topics of conversation.

"I'm not smoking," she says. "I found a pack in my purse and had the aide throw it out. Then I remembered a pack upstairs and had the aide get it and throw it out too."

I am floored.

Betty felt a great sense of identification with other smokers, thrown out of buildings, like the homeless huddled on the streets, puffing and littering. I couldn't enter her house because the particulates choked me. When I had asked her in the past why she kept smoking she said, "Smoking is one of my few pleasures in life."

Now I ask, "How come you quit *now?*"

"I want to have a chance to live in the house that Penny's building," she says. "If I smoke, I won't have that chance. Not smoking slows down the emphysema process."

I wonder how she's finally gotten the message—and from where. The web?

"Betty, we did all the paperwork, but we forgot one thing you wanted done," I say on my Sedona phone. "You wanted an ethical will."

"Don't feel the need."

"Don't feel the *need*?" I repeat. An ancient practice, ethical wills are a spiritual counterpart to the legal documents, a way of passing on one's blessings, hopes, and values—telling others what mattered to you, what moved you.

"I don't feel any impulse. I don't feel the need."

"Why?"

"Good question." Pause. "This may be truly arrogant, but I've lived an ethical life and that's the model, so there's little or no need to write an ethical will. . . . It is impossible to know what is next."

"So your *life* is the ethical will?"

"Exactly!"

What am I doing? Interviewing her? Collecting data?

Friday, October 28

Ernest and I are back from Sedona, jet-lagged, tired, and happy.

"Oh, I'm glad you're back," Betty says, answering my phone call. Her voice sounds rough and she is coughing.

"How're things going?" I ask. This has become my routine question, my way of both asking and keeping my distance, objectifying and confirming Betty's preferred vision: Things happen to her.

"This has been a very hard day," she says, struggling to catch her breath.

"I'm sorry."

"I'll probably have to go back to the hospital."

"I'm sorry."

"Can you read me the stuff—the obituary and memorial service arrangements we wrote? I need to know it now."

"Let me find it." I fumble through the stacks of papers I'd left on my desk when I went to Sedona. "I thought Penny would bring you her copy when she came for your birthday," I say. I am making that up, making conversation, covering my ineptitude. Her life is misplaced on my desk.

"Here you are," I say lightly. "Should I read it?"

"If you don't mind." Her voice is almost a whisper.

"You might want some of this changed," I say, settling on the couch with pen and paper.

"'Betty Frankel Kirschner died after being screwed around for five years by a variety of illnesses. . . .'"

Betty laughs. "Is that what I said?"

"I couldn't make that up, Betty. Everyone laughs when they hear it." I don't add they think it sounds like her, captures her anger and feelings of being acted upon. "Shall I change it to 'died after dealing with a variety of illnesses'?"

"That's better," she says hesitantly.

We review the memorial service plans. Yes, that's right, a Reform or Reconstructionist rabbi. Yes, that's right, the Prayer of Remembrance, Kaddish in English and Hebrew. And yes, that's right, no mention of Israel.

"What an imposition on Bonnie," Betty says. "Having my memorial service at her house."

"Bonnie said she'd be honored," I say. "She wants to do it. She'll follow your wishes."

"Okay. . . . Thanks, Laurel." Her voice is very heavy.

"I'll fix up the papers tomorrow, mail them, and call you."

"Yes, tomorrow."

Saturday, October 29

Betty almost never leaves a message on my answering machine, but while I am at my "Liquid Balance" water aerobics class, she does leave the briefest of brief messages. She says she's "feeling better." I surmise that she wants the papers mailed out to her today, so I prepare them, print three copies—one for me, one for Penny, and one for her. I put mine in a new turquoise folder labeled "Betty," and put each of the others in an envelope with a LOVE stamp.

It's a perfect fall day—temperature in the 60s, sun, no wind, blue sky, and trees alight with oranges, reds, and yellows. Brown leaves crunch under my feet as I walk to the post office to mail my letters. I kick into piles of yellow leaves raked to the curb. How good it is to be alive.

"Hi, Betty." I call her from my cell phone on the way back from the post office. "Wanted you to know that I've just mailed your papers. How're things going?"

"Better. I called Penny right after we talked yesterday. The service can't be at Bonnie's. It's just too much of an imposition. I told Penny just rent a room at the Kent Student Union."

I feel had.

Sunday, October 30

"I told Penny I don't want any more interventions," Betty tells me on the phone.

"You need to be in hospice then," I say.

"No. I want to be at home with *my* Dr. Lee." Dr. Lee is an osteopath with no license to practice in any of Ohio's hospitals. She's in a solo practice and has no secretary or nurse. She makes house calls. Recently she's been training to become a missionary. Penny thinks she's a quack. "I've had a long talk with Dr. Lee," Betty says. "I want to be with her."

"Then Dr. Lee has to be your emergency contact number. Otherwise you'll be brought back to the hospital and resuscitated or intubated."

"We're working that out," Betty says.

"Everyone does have the right to choose how they want to go," I say. "Yes."

I believe Betty has chosen doctor-assisted suicide—illegal in Ohio—and that she believes Dr. Lee will comply.

Monday, October 31

"You sound funny," Betty says. She's called to thank me for a greeting card I sent her from Sedona.

"Oh, I'm just writing," I equivocate. I don't tell her that I'm writing about her dying. "Let me go onto the couch where I'll be away from the writing energy." I take my Daybook with me.

"I love the card, but even more I love what you wrote," she says.

"What did I write?"

"'Dear Betty, Thank you. You have given me so much, including the beauty of Sedona. As I drive around I say your name and it is taken by the wind and inscribed in the rocks.'"

My eyes tear. I think hers do too.

"How're things going?" I ask.

"Feeling good enough to feel bored," she answers. Over the years, when her agoraphobia acted up and she complained of boredom, I would suggest she make political phone calls or become a phone buddy for a shut-in—to do something she'd consider of value and useful from her house. "But," she would say, "I can't trust that I'd do it."

"I'm sure not bored today," I say. "Autumn's sensuousness is everywhere."

"The problem with happiness is you don't know you have it till it's gone," she says. "I read that somewhere."

"So when were you happy?"

"Going down Oak Creek Canyon from Flagstaff to Sedona."

"Have you got your wheelchair yet?"

"And my walker. It would be good to get halfway around my house." She laughs. "Then where'd I be?"

"Halfway around," I say.

"Maybe I'll go on the porch and breathe the air."

"How're the aides working out?"

"The daytime ones are wonderful. The night one is awful. She's scared of everything."

"Like?"

"Like the stop sign at the end of the street."

I remember the many times when Betty would not leave her house because she was afraid of that stop sign, afraid her car would be unable to stop, certain it wouldn't in the snow. She canceled our plans to meet so often that we began to hedge our plans with caveats, "If it's not snowing or going to snow or has snowed."

Betty is starting to cry. "All I've been thinking about is getting to live in the new house Penny's building for me. And then I had this sudden thought that the house will be full of allergens. And I will be so sick. It's awful. I won't be able to breathe."

After we hang up, I finish my unpacking and find one of the little presents I had bought for Betty in Sedona, a tiny silver Kokopelli charm. The Hopi flute player and guide has been one of her icons. I pull a length of rainbow ribbon, long enough to slip over her head, onto the charm. I append a note, "This is to carry with you." I remove the note, fearful she'll think I mean "carry it with you when you die." Then I reattach it. Maybe I do mean that.

NOVEMBER

Tuesday, November 1

I twisted my foot yesterday and feel the telltale signs of plantar fasciitis.
The cure is to stay off my foot and do my toe agility and red resistance-
band exercises. Today I woke up at eleven and stayed in bed for another
half hour. I decided not to take a shower, wash my hair, or get dressed.
I am not going to call anyone or do anything I don't want to do. I am
taking a sick day.

I've stopped teaching at The Ohio State University, and I draw my
pension. But I can't say I am actually retired. I don't want to say it either.
Indeed, in February and March I will be a Distinguished Fellow at the
University of Melbourne in Australia. On the way home I'll vacation in
Tahiti.

I am not retired. Instead, I'm taking a sick day. I am at my computer
in my makeshift pajamas, paisley robe, and mismatched house slippers. I
am going to write all day if I want to.

I think about Betty's year-long sick days. On her worst days
she would curl up into her swivel chair, tethered to her oxygen tank,
watching endless reruns of the news and weather reports, and smoking.

"Do you turn the oxygen off when you're smoking?" I asked her once.
She said, "You don't think I'm nuts, do you?"

On her best days, over this past year, someone might drive her to lunch, a party, a doctor's appointment, or to the rehabilitation center, where she would join others for a brief lecture on healthy habits before working out on the treadmill and stationary bike, aiming for a five-minute stint. A nurse would take her blood pressure before, during, and after each exercise station. Rescue personnel would stand by.

"What I can't understand," Betty would often say to me, "is that there are all these fat people here. Cardiac patients. Diabetics. And they don't stop eating junk food."

Hello.

"I feel better after the exercise," she would tell me, adding, "I never thought I'd say something like that." Betty dislikes feeling her heart pump or her skin sweat.

Rarely has Betty phoned her friends this year. She waits for them to call, even though she feels "bored and angry." "People can't deal with chronic illness," she explains. I think she's depressed.

I contrast how I am spending my "sick day" with how Betty has been spending her "sick days." I am writing and working out my feelings about Betty's illness. I am trying to heal my foot. I am not blaming anyone but my overzealous self for the plantar fasciitis. Well, don't I feel superior! I sit in my smugness for a bit. But there is a world of difference between acute and chronic problems.

The phone rings.

"Hi, Mom. It's me, Ben."

"Hi. What's up?" I ask. "I've been thinking about you." Last week, my older son, Ben, had spinal surgery to fuse two of his neck vertebrae. He's wearing a neck brace and is on sick leave for three weeks.

"I want to talk about Josh," Ben says. "I'm concerned."

My younger son, Josh, has had a chronic back problem for the last two years. He's been unable to work, and the Ohio Bureau of Workman's Compensation, due to internal audit problems, will not settle his claim until March, two and one-half years after the injury. In the meantime Josh cannot seek gainful employment and is not entitled to disability benefits. His physical pain has been augmented by the colon cancer of his father and the breakup of his four-year, live-in relationship with Lisa.

"Josh is dispirited," I say. "Maybe give him a call."

"Okay, I'll do that," Ben says. "Bye. I love you."

"I love you too."

When Josh was six he discovered his father's liquor stash. When he was sixteen, he went into treatment for alcoholism. Twenty-five years of sobriety later, he is still fearful of the possible effects of prescription painkillers and antidepressants. He spends much of his time in a virtual world, playing "Ever Quest," a real-time Internet game where he is a Game Master. "The game is saving my sanity," he told me.

What I think is really saving his "sanity" is Akiva, his ten-year-old son, my only grandson. But I fear that the longer Josh's disability lasts, the more likely his ex-wife will sue for sole custody. Sometimes I feel I haven't done enough for Josh, and sometimes I feel that I've done too much by helping him financially. Josh's chronic problems have created a chronic problem for me.

Betty is the one friend who knows Josh's story from his childhood to his parenthood, from my divorce to his divorce. Although I had not planned on talking to her today, I phone her.

"This is not particularly nice to say," Betty says, "but maybe the threat of losing Akiva will be a wake-up call for Josh."

I like hearing Betty play "Laurel"—finding the upbeat in the downbeat. I feel better.

"How're you doing?" I ask.

"Hives. I have these horrible hives," she answers. "All over my body. I start itching around four in the afternoon and I itch until four in the morning. They really hurt too."

"Anything new in your diet? Meds?"

"No. I'm on more steroids to see if that will stop the pain."

"Are hives related to emphysema?"

"No."

"You've quit smoking, and maybe the toxins are coming out," I say.

"I hadn't thought of that."

"You're supposed to be in water a lot when you quit smoking," I say, looking for a solution.

"That's something I can't do."

"Why not?"

"I can't breathe in the shower. Or in the tub when I let the water run."

"Maybe check the web?"

I retire to bed with Fodor's guide to Australia.

Thursday, November 3

For five years, my memoir writing group has met bimonthly on Thursday afternoons. We are eight women in our fifties, sixties, and seventies. Since we started meeting together, one member has completed her M.F.A. and two have published books. The more time we spend together, the more intimate we have become.

Today I read from my Daybook about Betty, me, and the end of life. Erica, who volunteers at hospice, tells us, "One of the advantages of hospice is that they know how the dying process progresses. They can read the signs and alert the family. About two weeks before death, they can see the changes."

"Is that true for pulmonary diseases too?" I ask.

"Mostly true for cancer patients."

"My father doesn't want to go into hospice," says Bev. Her ninety-eight- year-old father lives in a nursing home. "My father's standing up now. They said he'd never walk again, but he's going to."

"I don't know what I'd choose to do," Nancy says. She's our oldest member. Infusions reduce her rheumatic pain.

"Do any of us?" Deanne asks in her gravelly voice. She has chronic bronchitis.

"Modern medicine wants us to live forever," Linda T. says. She takes care of her eighty-five-year-old stepfather.

"My greatest fear is that I'll get caught up in that system," Erica says, "despite knowing better!"

"It's the hypocrisy that really bothers me," I blurt out. "For example, doctor-assisted suicide. It's illegal in Ohio. Why would you ask your doctor to do that, risk her license? Just do it yourself, if that's what you want."

"I don't think I'd have the energy," says Deanne.

"Well, there are morphine suppositories," Diana says. She's our youngest member.

"I'm allergic to morphine," Deanne says.

We all laugh.

"What about driving your car into a light pole?" I ask.

"Your family would get the insurance," Linda R. says. She belongs to an investment club.

My mother's death was a doctor's mercy killing after her cancer metastasized to her bones and her brain. I think my father was murdered.

Tuesday, November 8

It's my father's birthday. If he were alive, he'd be 107 years old. Ever since I began writing about Betty, Father's been in my dreams. In one dream I am carrying a heavy burden when Father appears beside me. His chest is caved in, his arms and legs are emaciated, he moves haltingly, shoulders hunched forward, protecting his heart. "Look how much of a burden I am carrying," he says.

No one expected my mother to predecease my father, but she did. For forty years she lived with second-hand smoke from his four-packs-of-Parliaments-a-day habit.

Wednesday, November 9

"How're you doing?" I ask Betty. She is still at home in Kent.

"I've gotten my stubbornness back and I'm babying myself," she says. She's on massive steroids and her voice sounds heavy and deep.

"What're you doing?" I ask, again.

"Little things."

"Like what?"

"Just little things, that's all."

"Like what?" I use my lilting voice.

"Too embarrassing even to mention."

"Oh? Like what?" I use my consoling voice. I wait silently for her to answer my probe.

"Oh, ... taking a shower ..."

"Yes, and ..."

"... Oh, taking a walk around the house."

These are the same things she mentioned last week. What isn't she mentioning?

Why am I pushing her? Do I want more detail for my Daybook?

Thursday, November 10

"We don't know how you and Betty have remained friends," Bev says after I read again from my Daybook to the memoir writing group.

Nancy says, "Maybe if you tell us how you became friends, we'll understand better."

Friday, November 11

I call Betty. She's back in Robinson Memorial Hospital and will be there for a couple of weeks.

"Anything I shouldn't tell my memoir writing group about you or our friendship?" I ask Betty.

"You decide, Laurel."

Thursday, November 17

Betty and I met in New York City in August 1970 at the newly formed Sociology Women's Caucus. Over one hundred women gathered in a too-small meeting room in the Hilton Hotel. Betty stood up, commanded the floor, talking with her hands, and shaking her shoulder-length, glistening, prematurely white hair to emphasize points. When women stood up and applauded, her blue eyes sparkled.

After the caucus, Betty sat spine-straight on a hotel couch outside the meeting room—smoking. I joined her—smoking then too. Her badge said, "Kent State University," mine, "The Ohio State University." Most of the women at the caucus were from the East Coast. We were both outlanders.

We were both Jewish, me half so, on my mother's side, and we were both in our mid-thirties, tall and thin—Betty a little shorter and thinner than I was—and we were both wearing Anne Klein II designer clothes. Hers were wrapped tightly around her, as if her body needed them to hold it together. Mine were draped loosely, as if my body needed to move freely, unencumbered.

"I want to get my Ph.D.," Betty said.

"Come to Ohio State University," I said, outlining our post-M.A. program. "Work with me."

Betty came to OSU and joined a sterling cohort of young, single, and academically motivated women. She rented a basement apartment a mile from my home and commuted most weekends back to Kent to her then-husband, Joe, and two-year-old Penny.

These were academic times when intellectual alliances created friendships in the academy and when the status distinctions between faculty and graduate students were breached. The personal was the political, and the political generated academic research. The graduate students and I were jazzed. We formed a community and forged a new specialty, the sociology of gender. We dubbed one of the seminars "Never Ending." We all became friends. But Betty became my best friend. For thirty-five years we have been best friends.

"I don't know what this is under my arm," Betty said, midway through the autumn quarter. "But I need to have it removed. Can you take me to the hospital?" I did. The lump was not malignant.

After that, several times a week throughout that academic year, Betty and I would sit on my brown velvet couch, drinking tea, smoking, and talking about men and children and feminist causes and memories of our grandfathers and what it meant to be Jewish and arguing over whether people had any choice about what they did with their lives. I thought they did. She thought people had no agency, so whatever happened to them was not their fault. For her, determinism trumped free will.

Friday, November 18

"Hi. How'd the breath test go?" I ask.

"What we expected," Betty says.

"Sorry to hear that."

"We need to correct some stuff on the papers we wrote," Betty says. "I remember the name of the university where I taught a long time ago in Kansas: Washburn. Two of the best years of my life. Don't give Gerry the clothes. Get New Jersey names."

"Anything else?"

"Haven't finished reading it."

Saturday, November 19

My death and dying papers are not in order.
My death and dying papers are not in order.
My death and dying papers are not in order.
My death and dying papers are not in order.

Monday, November 21

I feel tired, old, sick, angry, testy, touchy, ready to club anyone who comes near. My entire body hurts. The flu. I am nasty to everyone and I don't care. If I am this awful when I am only temporarily ill, why should I come down so hard on Betty? Actually, I don't know how she does it—keeps up a front, or as she would say, "shows good behavior."

It's been at least five years since Betty has felt well. I remember the last time she was able to drive herself to Cuyahoga Falls for one of our weekends of ogling the wedding parties at the Sheraton Suites Hotel. A two-hour drive for me, twenty minutes for her. When she arrived, she looked healthier than I did. But she obsessed over her blood pressure and refused to leave the hotel because she felt "it was not a good idea to move around too much."

Betty wanted to watch *Crossing Over*, a TV series that featured a "medium" who claimed he could talk to the dead. At home she watched it four times a day. "It makes me feel closer to my father," she explained.

I wanted to talk about how bad I felt about taking early retirement from the sociology department and becoming an adjunct professor in the College of Education.

Betty stayed in the room watching *Crossing Over* while I walked to the nearby nearly deserted Riverfront district—antiques, art, and collectible stores with no customers. A Betty Boop tempted me but that store was closed. By the Eagles Club entrance there was a sign, "Don't even try to come in if you haven't paid your dues." A clean-cut, well-groomed man in surgical scrubs and tennis shoes stopped his pounding on the Eagles' plate-glass window, groaned, pulled his pants down, and squatted toward the pavement. Was he sick, drunk, an escapee from a mental hospital? He snaked away, his back toward me, to the parking lot and tried to break into a car. "If in doubt, call it out," my father had instructed me as a child. I went into a candy shop, used their phone, and called the police. The dispatcher asked for my name.

"Why?" I said.

"Just for the record," she said. "And your home address."

Later that day, Officer Dane came to the Sheraton Suites with an affidavit for me to sign. He had called my home and Ernest told him where I was staying.

"No," I said. "I won't sign. I'd have to come back up from Columbus to testify. . . . That's why people don't report things. . . . I can't say whether or not he was drunk."

"Well, he was very drunk," said Officer Dane. "We have him in jail, drying out. He's not happy."

"Why was he in scrubs?" I asked. "Was he a surgeon?"

Officer Dane avoided my questions.

"Well," I said, "if you got him, you don't need me."

"Well, by Ohio law you just said the words that get you off. I can't force you to testify."

"Thank goodness!"

"Just know that you've saved someone's life."

Already this year, in Sedona, I saved the life of an elderly man from an elderly woman's blind, back-up driving. Maybe my new role in life is to be a guardian angel.

Thursday, November 24

"Happy Thanksgiving, Betty," I say.

"The same to you."

"Has Penny arrived?"

"Yes, and Mike. Jack is adorable," she says. "I feel terrible that I can't do the Thanksgiving dinner like I used to do it."

"Will you go to Bonnie's?"

"If I can, we will. If not, someone will bring the food here."

"I remember a Thanksgiving at your house one year when your father came," I say.

Mr. Frankel, a white-haired, lean man, sat on the brown velvet couch that Betty and I had picked out, similar to mine. In a New Jersey accent he called to his daughter, cooking in the kitchen, "Betty, bring me some water! Betty, bring me some more ice! Betty, come on out here!" She did. He patted the cushion next to him and said, "Sit down, Betty." She did. He had been a cantor in his small synagogue, and now he burst forth into song, "Take me out to the ballgame . . ." Betty and her father were Dodgers fans. I felt like an interloper.

When I was a little girl, my dad would sing me to sleep in his scratchy Irish tenor, "Hush little baby, don't say a word, Papa's gonna buy you a mockingbird. If that mockingbird don't sing, Papa's gonna buy you a diamond ring . . ."

Now Betty says to me on the phone, "I remember that Thanksgiving. Daddy, bless him. He loved everything I did."

Saturday, November 26

When was it that Betty became seriously ill? I think it was in 1999, when she tried to quit smoking by going to a smoking cessation retreat in Pennsylvania. She quit smoking, came home, and had a "stroke." There was no brain damage, loss of speech or motor function. Nor was she admitted to the hospital. I think she had a panic attack. She began smoking again.

The experience tired and frightened her. She decided to go to Heritage House, an assisted-living facility in Delaware, to be near her daughter. I visited her there once, staying in assisted-living too.

"When you get ill, you lose your independence," I said. Betty and I sat on a bench outside Heritage House so Betty could smoke. I continued my thought, "Also lost is the sense of who you are because you aren't socializing with your community."

"That's exactly how I feel," she said. She squashed her Lark under a worn-out red slipper, retrieved the butt, shredded its half inch of unsmoked tobacco, twisted the paper around the shreds and the filter, and flicked the bundle over her shoulder onto a half-buried garden spade. "I feel my lives have disappeared."

"Did you say 'lives'?" I asked.

"My colleague friends. My political friends. My union friends. My Sedona friends. I'm not in those lives anymore. Heritage House is not my life." She lit another Lark.

A List of Approved Suppliers was posted on a nearby door. I nodded toward it, shook my head disapprovingly, and said, "We're sure living at a time when medical care is commodified." Betty's smoking had triggered one of my defense modes, thinking in sociological jargon.

"You're telling me?" she said.

"We have the runaway sludge of the health-care system and its tributaries, insurance-driven, for-profit hospitals, and overworked, underpaid floor staff." I was on a roll.

"You're telling me!"

I wanted to yell about her smoking, but I controlled myself and took the high road. I lectured at her. "When you enter the medical system, you enter an ongoing story. As a patient, you have almost no influence on the story's plot. You have no control. You're a prop—a blip on a monitor, a number on a chart, specimens in a tube, a computer printout."

Betty joined right in. "The medical doctors see me as body parts reduced to electronic body parts. The osteopaths see me as connected body parts reduced to graphs. So I've been to see a chiropractor. He's the first one to treat me as a whole person."

A chiropractor now?

"I feel better, and I feel the possibility of leaving Heritage House." Betty went on, "Years ago in Sedona, I bought myself a magic wand."

"I remember that," I said.

"You know, *Cinderella* and *The Wizard of Oz*, my favorite stories. Wave your magic wand and everything's okay."

Who waves the wand, Betty?

"That's been my story," Betty says, "looking for a miracle."

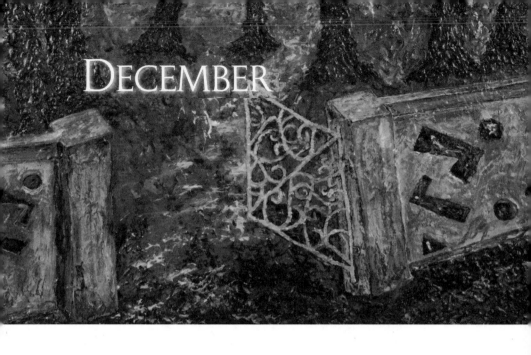

December

Thursday, December 1

I haven't called Betty in a week, which is a record of sorts. I didn't want to walk about in her world. I was withdrawing, calling other friends. But I feel guilty, so I call her. She tells me that she is "recovering" and that she has been outside and driven herself around the corner to the Burger King to get a Coke. When she says, "I feel as if I've done something," I can hear anger toward me in her voice. "Do you realize how hard it is for me to be outside and not smoke?"

"You associate smoking with the *outdoors*?"

"I associate everything but my *house* with smoking!"

What!?! I associate every room in her house and everything in her house with her smoking.

Three years ago, Penny and Mike were driving from Delaware to install new bathroom fixtures for Betty. "Would you come to Kent and help me pick them out?" she asked.

Of course.

Rain poured down that Wednesday in early May on the roads and the yellow barrels that lined them for miles, and the normal two-hour drive stretched to three. I arrived at Betty's house tired, angry, and needing to pee.

"Where've you been?" she asked accusingly. "I'm hungry. I've made reservations at the Kent Holiday Inn."

My lungs filled up immediately with the smoke and particulates that floated about her house. I coughed, my eyes watered, and my nose stung. She'd been smoking a couple packs of Larks a day in that house for the past thirty-three years.

"Let's get lunch," I wheezed. "And let's sit in the nonsmoking section." We entered my first new car in ten years, a white retro-styled Chrysler 300M. "How do you like my new car?"

"It looks like an egg," Betty said, fastening her seatbelt. She is allergic to eggs.

"Look at the clock!" I said. It's an old-fashioned round one, with hands.

Silence.

"Leather seats," I said.

Silence.

"Genuine California walnut trim." My hand glided over the steering wheel. "Not plastic."

Silence.

"There are four Bose speakers." Betty loves music.

Silence.

"It reminds me of when I was a kid in my dad's fancy cars," I soldiered on. "And at the same time I feel like I'm an elegant grown-up lady."

Betty said, "It would be better if it had a clock."

"It does have a clock, Betty."

"A *real* clock," Betty said. "A *digital* one."

After lunch we went to the "nearby" Lowe's to look for fixtures, which took more than a half hour of stop-and-go traffic. We spent an hour talking to the clerk figuring out what would fit in Betty's bathroom. I felt exhausted from the plastics out-gassing in the store.

"Did I tell you," Betty said on our half-hour journey to the motel, "that Penny and Mike are not coming to put in the bathroom?"

"What?"

We checked into a nonsmoking room at the Holiday Inn and

took naps. After dinner I said, "Want me to read my new piece about Sedona?" Reading my writing to her had been a regular ritual during our times together. I'd settle on my bed with my pen and new writing on my lap, and Betty would say, "Just a minute. Let me get a pencil and paper." Then she'd settle on her bed while I read and she jotted notes about what didn't make sense or didn't work or didn't scan. Helpful notes. If she had written something, we'd reverse roles. We trusted each other as first listeners.

"Maybe later," Betty said. "It's time for *American Idol.*"

"What?"

"I told you about *American Idol.*"

"You said it was Tuesday night. This is Wednesday."

"Did I? Well it's Tuesday night and Wednesday night too."

I hunkered down to watch my first *American Idol.* The program had as much interest to me as a middle-school talent show. I hadn't seen my "best friend" in seven months. I was ticked.

When the commercial came on I said, "Let me show you my new photos." Sharing trip photos had also been one of our rituals.

"I need a cigarette," Betty said. "Want to join me outside?"

"I'll just read my novel."

American Idol came to an end. I took a big breath. "I've been thinking about my shadow side," I said.

"Yes?"

"This might be painful."

"Go ahead . . ."

"In some ways you *are* my shadow."

Betty, you are becoming the person I fear I will become: self-centered, slothful, sick.

"I'm not surprised," she said. "I've become my own shadow."

On the drive home the next day I was sad and angry. Did I ever want to see her again? When I arrived home, I complained to my husband, Ernest. He said, "Betty's *family.*"

This was three years ago.

Today on the phone I say, "Hey, Sister Betty, I'm so proud of you for quitting smoking! Good for you!"

Monday, December 6

Betty loves having tea, alone or with others. The heart-shaped tea napkins with the logo "Betty & Co." I sent her have arrived. "People laugh when they see them," she says. She doesn't thank me, which surprises and saddens me.

Saturday, December 10

Betty calls me at 9:30 a.m. from her home, unusual both that she is calling and that's she is calling that early. I've just rolled out of bed and I'm making my coffee.

"Have you got a minute?" she asks.

"What's up?" I ask, concerned.

"I want to tell you a dream I had." In the dream she is in a cave with her ex-husband, Joe. There's an earthquake, a terrorist attack, and workmen banging on the plumbing. She tells Joe, "We have to get out of here." But he is on the floor, his head a bleeding snake head.

"So how do you interpret it?" I ask.

"Another person who has abandoned me," she says.

"You sound very angry at Joe."

"I'm furious."

Betty says Joe hasn't asked her about her health or hospitalizations.

Monday, December 12

"My legs are getting fat and my arms and my face," Betty says. She's still at home. Last week the pulmonologist gave her a massive steroid shot that has made her ravenously hungry. "When I talk about how fat I am, people say I'm an anorectic. I weigh 112 pounds now—more than I've ever weighed in my life." When I met Betty, she was five feet, eight inches tall and weighed 102 pounds. Now she's perhaps four inches shorter.

"I've put on a lot of weight, even without steroids," I say. "We look okay to others, but we just don't feel like ourselves."

"That's exactly right," she says.

"It's probably good, though, that you have a little extra weight."

"Good for *what?* For the next incident?"

"Hi, Betty," I say. She's back in Robinson Memorial Hospital. "My turn to tell a dream."

"Good," she says. "Break my boredom."

"In my dream I'm with a busload of Unitarians."

"Ugh," Betty grunts.

I had asked her once why she had such distaste for Unitarians. She said they had "taken away" her friends, turning them into something they weren't, and providing them with a community from which she was excluded, albeit by choice. She has felt abandoned by friends and lovers. She cried when I told her I had joined the Unitarian Church choir. She refused to listen to the choir's CD of the *Magnificat.* She railed when she learned a Unitarian minister would perform her daughter's marriage ceremony.

I continue telling her my dream. "The bus stops at an old boyfriend's house. His mother takes me into the basement where she profusely apologizes for her anti-Semitic behavior toward me, blaming it on her husband. 'I was only a secretary who married up,' she says. We hug and reminisce. When I come up from the basement, the busload of Unitarians has gone off without me."

"Good thing too," Betty responds.

"The Unitarians and I are not going in the same direction anymore," I say, realizing that for these moments, at least, one of the gulfs between Betty and me has been bridged.

I continue, "I sense anti-Semitism in the church now."

"No more than anywhere else," she says.

If we were to continue this conversation, I know she would blame Israel and American Jews for the anti-Semitism. She is entirely sympathetic to the Palestinians, enraged at the Israelis. She holds Jews to higher standards than other people.

Some Jews, I've come to think, form their identity around an ideal of unimpeachable virtue. Betty is one of them. If Jews should kill those who are killing them, they would kill their heritage of moral superiority. To respond to terrorism with violence is worse than the terrorism. I've been afraid to push her, but in my heart I think she thinks, "A dead Jew with clean hands is better than a live Jew with dirty ones."

Whenever news of crimes came over the radio, her father would wail, "*Gott in Himmel.* Let it not be a Jew." It was not the assailed he was wailing about, but the assailant. "What will *they* do to *all of us Jews,* if one of us robs or murders?" he intoned. Betty still expresses relief when the perpetrator of a heinous crime is not a Jew, or at least does not have a Jewish-sounding name.

How horrible it must be to carry the weight of your people on your shoulders—and then to find those people lacking! If I felt that way, I think I would be depressed—and sick—all the time.

Saturday, December 24

Christmas is Betty's least favorite holiday. She can neither join the festivities nor ignore them. Everyone, she feels, is having a party to which she is not invited.

Once I did invite her to take part in my Christmas Eve tradition. My sons and I arrived at our neighbor's as dark was falling and the neighbor man was bringing in a scraggly tree, purchased cheap so the seller could get it off his lot. We decorated it with kid-made ornaments, tin tinsel, and angel hair, exchanged token presents, ate a traditional Swedish dinner, sang, drank schnapps, and wished each other "a very merry Christmas." Then Betty arrived, wearing jeans and a sweatshirt, bearing no gifts. She complained about the "ugly lights," "grotesque spade-shaped Santas," and "holiday cheer" that "bombarded" her on her drive down from Kent. I was embarrassed and ashamed.

I still don't understand how the season can be such a problem for her. Maybe it's because in her mind it is not just a party to which she is not invited—it's a whole season.

Tonight I call her at her home. "Happy Hanukkah," I say. The two holidays are on the same day this year. "How're you doing?"

"Can you believe it?" she says. "I was able to get to downtown Kent to have lunch with Bonnie and everything was frickin' closed. It was noon. On Christmas Eve Day. Not even Christmas yet."

Kent is a university town and the students have gone home for the winter break. I am thinking it's nice that the storekeepers are giving their employees and themselves a little break too.

"So did you find somewhere to have lunch?" I ask.

"Bob Evans. But it was too crowded."

I groan.

I've done something completely different this Christmas Eve, but I won't tell Betty about it. Ernest and I went to Ernest's daughter and son-in-law's Evangelical megachurch, Xenos, to hear their children, Natasha and Katya, sing in the children's choir. When we arrived at 3:30 for the 4 o'clock service, the thousand-seat Fellowship Hall was almost full with clean-cut young families. Three huge television monitors were suspended above the proscenium stage. Different bands played, quartets and sextets sang, adult choirs sang, children sang, children danced, everyone sang, and Christian rappers rapped. A preteen girl introduced a reading from the New Testament, an older woman introduced a reading from the Old Testament. The adult education coordinator, a physician, came up on stage, wearing a red polo shirt, khakis, and Nikes.

"How difficult the holiday season is for so many," he said into his shirt-mike. "I see so much turmoil and problems in my medical practice at this time." He paused, then continued, "I used to be in turmoil too because I didn't know—until I found Xenos—that if I took Jesus as my personal savior, my sins would be forgiven, my place in heaven assured."

There is an expectant hush in the audience.

"This is the lesson—and the present—of Christmas," he concludes.

The audience claps. I think he's preaching to the choir, but then I realize he's preaching to those of us who haven't chosen Jesus.

After the service we celebrate at Ernest's daughter's house. An old and worn angel from Ernest's childhood tops the tree.

Sunday, December 25

I love Christmas because I don't have to food shop, cook, or clean. Ben and his wife, Tami, have everyone over for ham, beans, and salads. Their daughter, Shana, makes brownies. We take turns opening presents, most of which have come from my sister, Jessica, and her husband, John.

A family of three came to Betty's house with finger food from

Greek and Italian restaurants in Akron. "That wasn't what I was expecting," she tells me on the phone. "I was hoping for turkey and all the works. Or roast beef and all the works."

This family has honored Betty's abhorrence of all things Christmas. Why doesn't Betty see that?

"I made the mistake of telling my neighbor that my computer wasn't working right and I had to spend an hour sitting next to him while he tried to fix it," she continued.

"Did he?"

"No. I got tired, and I had to ask him to leave."

"That's too bad."

"There are two good parties coming up—New Year's Eve and New Year's brunch—and I probably won't be able to go to either of them."

"It's nice to be invited, though."

Silence.

"What about Penny and Jack?" I ask. "How was their Christmas?" Betty has refused to go to her daughter's before Christmas because she doesn't want to be part of "whatever is going on there." *You don't have to take part,* I have said to her repeatedly. *Excuse yourself. You have an excuse. You're sick. You're tired.*

"They were at Mike's relatives' house," she says.

My call waiting beeps.

"Any idyllic notions I had about how my life would be in Delaware have been shattered," she says.

"Oh?"

"Jack's presents!"

"Yes?"

"Someone gave him a bow and arrow. And a BB gun."

When we hang up, I ask Ernest whether an eight-year-old boy should have a BB gun.

"That's the age I was," Ernest says. "In two years, they'll get him his first .22-caliber. Jack can help them pick it out."

Sometimes the contrast between Ernest and Betty startles me.

I pick up my phone message: "Grandma. It's me, Akiva. I love the piano keyboard you and Grampa got me for Christmas. It's great. It can play all the instruments. And songs. And you can even use it with videos—special effects. Listen to the song I wrote . . ."

A haunting melody in a minor key with chromatic modulation enters my ears. I want to cry.

"I call it 'Akiva's House of Many Rooms,'" he says.

Thursday, December 29

My granddaughter, Shana, and I are shopping the post-holiday sales at Easton. We have our shopping routines—criticize the clothes, browse the cosmetics, try on the hats, and then head for the sale racks. Today Shana happily finds New Year's gifts for her friends in Japan, Greece, and New York. No decision-dissonance for her. I can't help but contrast her joy with Betty's anguish over selecting gifts. It is not because Betty is ungenerous but because she "can't imagine what might please" whomever. So she comes empty-handed to parties and beats herself up over not sending people presents.

Yet the gifts Betty has sent me over the past thirty-five years have pleased me: "best-friend" socks; "sisters" pin; a butterfly-embossed hand mirror; a Death Valley T-shirt that changes colors in the sunlight; a little brass goddess; "Miriam"—an Ellis Island Collection doll wearing a little Jewish star and carrying a violin; and Ellen Goodman and Patricia O'Brien's book *I Know Just What You Mean: The Power of Friendship in Women's Lives.*

"Betty gave me a fine lace handkerchief for catching my tears at Ben and Tami's wedding," I tell Shana when we stop for lunch at Nordstrom. "I gave it back to her for Penny's wedding, and she gave it back to me for Josh's."

"Awesome," Shana says.

"And I'll use it at your wedding. . . . And if you have a child, at hers. . . ."

"Awesome, Grandma."

Friday, December 30

All week I have been sick with a cold or allergies, I'm not sure which. I had planned to drive up to Kent during the week to see Betty, but I have lacked the essential energy to even get out of bed. I have not called Betty all week. Nor has she called me. Am I learning to live without her?

Saturday, December 31

"Hi," I say to Betty. "I've been sick all week. Allergies. Ernest has taken up the carpet in the bedroom. That'll help."

"I wondered if you weren't sick," she says.

Why didn't you call me then?

"You don't sound so good yourself," I say.

"I almost died this week."

Why didn't she call me then?

"I am not going to make it," she says. "I want to live long enough to see Penny's new house, but I am not going to make it. Poor Penny. I cried for an hour on the phone."

Why didn't Penny call me?

"Do you think you should go into the hospital now for a few days?"

"They can't do anything for me."

"They can pound your chest, give you Ativan, put you on the CPAP breathing machine. Give your body a little rest."

"They can't do anything for me," she repeats.

Does she mean they can't help her live? Or they can't help her die?

"I'm a little better today," she says. "But I've gained twenty-five pounds. My thighs are hitting. My arms are like bowling pins. My cheeks are puffed out."

"You're probably holding water."

"Dr. Lee has put me on water pills."

"Good," I say.

"On top of everything else, Dr. Lee has closed her practice in Kent. She just told me yesterday. She'll be doing missionary medicine."

Betty's Dr. Lee brings her patients chicken soup.

"What a terrible loss for you," I say.

"I can't stop crying."

On January 7 Betty is moving to Delaware to be with her daughter. On February 8 I travel to Australia for six weeks. Will we ever see each other again?

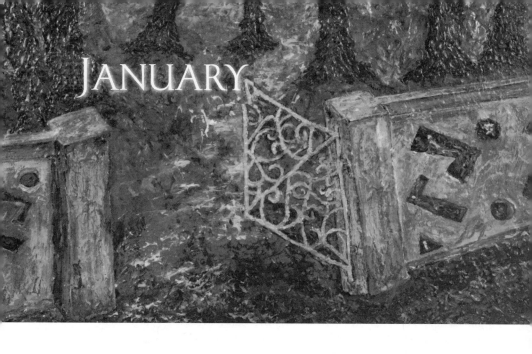

JANUARY

Sunday, January 1

A New Year. It's a beautiful warm and sunny day. I'm up early. I phone Betty and say, "I'm going to drive up to Kent if you're up to having company."

"Oh! This makes me cry," she says. "No. It'll be too much."

"... Okay.... I understand," although I don't. "So about your Dr. Lee leaving her practice in Kent. What a loss!"

"She'll keep me as a patient. She'll answer her cell phone immediately when I call," Betty says. "She'll be in Kent today. I'll call her cell and invite her over for tea."

Will they be negotiating Betty's doctor-assisted suicide? She can see Dr. Lee but not me! I feel rejected, relieved, angry, confused, and bitter. How can so many conflicting emotions coexist?

"Oh, by the way, Happy New Year," she says.

"You too."

Wednesday, January 4

Last night was not restful. My tooth hurt, my head hurt—both temples. Ernest's screeching two-level (BiPAP) sleep apnea machine woke me, a rattling on the stairs woke me, and Mimi-the-cat scrambling to the bedside table woke me. At 3 a.m. I took two sublingual melatonin tabs. At 11 a.m. I got out of bed, giving me just enough time to eat breakfast, take my fiber, and shower before my 12:20 mammogram.

The external disturbances were not the only cause of my sleeplessness. There were internal ones too. I had told myself I would start preparing my Australian workshops and lectures today even though I lack the inspiration to do so. It's work and I am tired and don't want to work anymore, although I do want the work-related perks, like the free travel, housing, and food that will be provided to Ernest and me in Australia.

Then my mind circles about all the people in my life with illnesses—my son Josh, recovering from a back injury; my son Ben, recovering from his neck surgery; my brother-in-law, John, surviving with a pacemaker, feeling "punk"; my friend John, surviving on one kidney, recovering from head injuries incurred by falling off a ladder; my friend Donald, recovering from brain surgery; and my friend Carla, facing the same.

Mammograms always make me nervous.

And, of course, there's Betty. I called her yesterday in the morning, but no one was home. I worried a bit, not too much, just a bit. I finally reached her in the late afternoon. She was feeling, she said, no worse than she had on New Year's Day, the day she had rejected my offer to visit her. She has felt well enough to go to her clinic for her ten minutes of exercise. I feel as if I am on a yo-yo string, brought up and sent down. Betty is holding the string.

In two days Penny and Mike will drive from Dover, Delaware, to Kent, Ohio, in their new truck. They will pack Betty's chosen things into it. Will she choose the watercolor of Sedona I painted that she asked me to give her? Will she choose the Sedona wall charm Ernest made that she asked him to give her? Mike will drive the truck back, while Penny will drive Betty's 1998 Taurus. Betty will take a sleeping pill for the six-hour trip. I may never see her again. *I may never see her again.*

Betty cried when she told me not to come up to Kent. Does she think we'll never see each other again too? If I were to come up to Kent, that truth too painful to be exposed would be exposed. We're both playing the yo-yo game.

I tell Ernest some of these thoughts. "Who knows," he says, "she might outlive us all."

Two days ago, driving and finding no talk radio I could stand listening to, I turned on my car's CD player, even though I knew better. Music distracts me. I go into the notes and follow their lead. I randomly clicked 3. "*I am there inside your mind,*" the Phantom sings, and I sing along with him . . . *inside my mind.* . . . I am on the 315 North freeway going faster and faster, passing a small COTA "mainstream" bus for the disabled probably going the speed limit. My heart thumps, keeping time with the music. Beautiful. I am going 85. Then already, so soon, here's my turn, the westbound outer belt, a 25 mph cloverleaf. I steer my Chrysler 300M onto the ramp, but the car slews off onto the embankment, into a furrow of mud and slop. I don't think I'll die here, but the car might turn over and I'll have to call Ernest and explain and have him come get me and he'll give me hell for being so careless and I'll never live it down ever. The car does not turn over but makes an odd sound, like bear claws clawing as I gun it up the other side of the embankment onto the ramp, and the outer belt. When I look back, the COTA mainstream bus is a few cars lengths behind. I was lucky this time. I turn the power button off. The Phantom dies.

Thursday, January 5

I want to ask Betty a lot of questions, but I can't make myself do it because I am questioning my motives. Did I want to go to Kent to see Betty, say good-bye, or have material for this Daybook? Have I become a writing vulture, like Truman Capote, picking the bones of my friend before she dies? Or am I dealing with her dying the way I habitually deal with any emotional issue—through writing?

"Do you have Penny's phone number?" I ask Betty.

"We'll have the same phone number," she says.

"Just one phone line?" I ask, incredulous. Betty's lifeline has been her telephone. Will she be able to plan a suicide without eavesdroppers? How will she have any phone privacy? How will I?

"Do you know Penny's e-mail?" I ask.

"I don't. But I'll probably use it. Mine isn't working."

No e-mail privacy either. What is Betty thinking?

"There's a lamp in the Coldwater Creek catalogue I might want for my table at Penny's," she says. "I wonder if it is too cute."

"Let me just look for it on the web. . . . Here it is." The lamp's a wrought iron tree with a bird and a nest in one of its branches. Ernest and I had considered that lamp for our back porch.

"It's very sweet," I say. "I like it."

"I'm going to order it then. Birds are a good theme for Delaware."

Twelve years ago, when I was flying from Chicago's Midway Airport, a seagull was sucked into an engine, and then a second seagull was sucked into a second engine. Thump! Thump! The pilot got on the PA system, told us what had happened, and said that he'd land us safely. For the next I-don't-know-how-many minutes, the plane circled low over Lake Michigan jettisoning fuel. No one in the plane acted frantic, the way they do in the movies. Some talked about their loved ones, others remained quiet and calm, accepting our fate, which turned out to be a crash-prepared landing back where we started, Midway Airport, Chicago.

Now I ask Betty, "Do you remember twelve years ago, when two seagulls flew into my airplane's engines?"

"I think of that often," she says. And then tells her "side" of the story. "I was in Montana, at a retreat. I could feel your energy flying around the room. I called your home in a panic, but no one answered. Two birds flew by my window—odd birds, birds that didn't belong in Montana. I cried and cried, and felt so lonely because you were gone. Then the fear passed, and I knew you were all right."

Friday, January 6

"I'm calling to tell you how optimistic I am about going to Penny's," Betty says. "It's an adventure. And I haven't had one of those for a long time."

Saturday, January 7

The phone rings as Ernest and I are heading out the door for the symphony. Betty leaves a message on the answering machine: "Just wanted to let you know I'm here. The trip went very well. I rode mostly with Mike in the truck—the most comfortable seat I've ever ridden in. Penny's house looks lovely. Call me when you have a chance."

Sunday, January 8

"Hel-*lo*," Mike answers the phone.

"Betty, please," I say.

Mike's a dispatcher, and his deep baritone voice must be very soothing to callers, but he jars me by saying, "Betty doesn't live here." He's laughing.

"It's me, Laurel. This is the number Betty gave me." I am flummoxed.

"I'll walk the phone over to *her* place. We're going to the casino in a few minutes."

"Mom," he shouts. "It's Laurel." I am back in time to when my mother and my aunts required the "married-ins" to call them Mom: "No in-laws or out-laws in our family." There is something endearing about Mike—a six-foot-two, two-hundred-fifty pounder—calling mini-Betty Mom. It was his idea too. He asked her permission to do so, the way generations ago a man might have asked permission to marry.

Betty's voice sounds scratchy but lifted, if voices can be lifted. "Everyone here is so nice," she says. "It is so wonderful to be here. I don't think twenty minutes goes by without someone asking if they can do something for me. Mike hugged me and cried and said, 'I didn't think you'd make it here, Mom.'"

Penny and Mike are laughing in the background.

"Enjoy the casino!" I say.

Monday, January 9

Betty calls to praise and to complain. Her apartment has many windows and she can see long distances across the flatness of rural Delaware. There are droves of birds in flyovers and the sky is mostly cloudless. The living space is painted in yellows, her bedroom in blue. Penny's hand-me-down furniture fills the space. Mike's friends and relatives met her upon arrival, and within five minutes all her boxes and belongings had been transferred to the right rooms.

"I have never felt so unconditionally loved in my life," she says. "Plus, I won $60 at the casino last night."

She ticks off a list of problems—the driveway, lack of doorbells, phone jacks, cable access, toilet paper holder—but the list is short.

I am truly happy that she is happy there.

"I'd like to see it sometime," I say, thinking I might visit.

"I'll try to get you photos," she answers.

"Maybe you'll decide to sell your house in Kent."

"It could happen. But the summer here is miserable."

"You could come back to Kent for the summer, stay in assisted living, . . . see your friends. . . ."

I ask myself, *Why are you doing this? Giving advice? Solving problems before they're raised as problems?*

Tuesday, January 10

I have let the deadline for sending a paper to the sociology meetings pass. This will be the first year I have not presented a paper at the convention. I will not go. Not going is one of my ways of letting go and moving on toward—oh, dear—*retirement*.

Until perhaps ten years ago, Betty went to the sociology conventions too, and we'd share a room, spending half our time complaining about men, children, sociology, departments, yellow barrels on the roads, fashion mistakes, and our bodies' failings.

In Detroit Betty thought she "still had it" when a handsome man asked her where there might be some good jazz. But then he returned to his wife with the information. In New Orleans we staged a sit-in, integrating women into the hotel's men-only bar. In Chicago we visited Le Moyne, my elementary school. In Washington, D.C., Betty laughed at me as I unconsciously struck the poses of the sculptures on the Mall. In San Francisco we shopped till we dropped, and in Kansas City, when the hotel flooded and signs told us to "follow the yellow . . . tapes," we co-wrote a poem about sexism at the convention. Later we published a satirical article based on that poem.

But what we did in New York City twenty-five or more years ago still sends shivers up my spine. My colleague Zhao had a brother, Wen, who was about to open a Chinese restaurant in the World Trade Center. Wen invited six of us to a private preopening dinner. We arrived by taxi around eight o'clock. Wen served us house specialty drinks for the next three hours. I'm not sure if we ate anything or not. We staggered out into a rainy night. In front of the building an oversized American flag was flagging in the rain. We decided to rescue it. We took the flag off the pole, folded it into makeshift triangles, hailed a cab, and brought ourselves and that flag back to the Hilton Hotel, where it ended up in Betty's and my room, and then in Betty's suitcase, and then back to Ohio, where she gave it to her handyman. I wonder if he still has it, and if Betty told him its provenance.

Friday, January 12

A call from a 702 area cell phone comes in. It's Penny. "How was Sedona?" she asks.

"Haven't we talked since October?" I say, surprised that we haven't.

"Guess not."

"I hear your new house is great."

"Yeah. We're happy."

Pause.

"Mom's in the hospital—the usual reasons: breathing, coughing, blood pressure, anxiety."

"I'm sorry," I say.

"She's not as bad as the last time, but she's told me again she doesn't want to be intubated. We'll have to get a bedside potty when she comes home. She can't walk the seven steps to her bathroom."

I call Betty at the confusingly named Kent General Hospital—Dover. Dover is in Kent County, Delaware. Her voice is hoarse, but she is awake and talkative. "Every EMT in Kent County arrived at my doorstep," she says. "They all know Mike. It was a cast of thousands."

"And you were the star of the show," I say.

"Yes! There was a little irony, though. Penny and Mike built the house without regard for an ambulance and designed a walkway unintended for a wheeled gurney. Getting to my ambulance was very bumpy, but it was full of friends. Mike knows everyone."

Betty arrived at Kent General with full troop support on Tuesday at 5:00 p.m. She was examined, given heavier doses of steroids, put on Xanax for anxiety, and sent home. Three blocks down the road Penny reversed course and brought her mother back to the ER. The doctor told Betty she was courageous to have left the ER but that it was right to return. Betty liked this doctor. For the next eighteen hours Betty remained in the ER, where a hanging sheet separated her bed from the others. There was a man with an accidental gunshot wound, an overdosed teenager, and a woman brought in for multiple Band-Aid-fixable mini stab wounds that she weekly inflicted on herself.

"When they got me a bed in my own room," Betty tells me, "three generations of Mike's family came and prayed over me."

"What did you do?" I imagine the flock of Christians flapping their angel wings.

"I'm very proud of myself. I told them to take it to someone who might like it better."

Her voice cracks. "These have been five of the best days of my elderly life," she says. "I am really happy, really loved being with Penny and Mike and Jack. I had five perfect days."

Saturday, January 14

"My muscles ache in my shoulders and arms," Betty says. She's still in the Kent General Hospital. "And I have hives again."

"Anxiety?" I ask.

"Maybe."

"But you are feeling better," I suggest.

"Some. . . . But this is the weirdest hospital. They close this unit every weekend and we all get moved somewhere else."

"Very weird!"

"Penny hangs out for hours," Betty says. "We've talked about doctors. Penny wants a doctor with all the science who tells her everything."

"Did you tell her what you want in a doctor?"

"I told her I want a doctor who cares about me as a human being, and pays attention to all my body parts as I talk about them."

"You're missing your own Dr. Lee, aren't you?"

"Yes, I am." Betty continues, "I dreamt that I was talking to Penny about Munchausen's-by-proxy. All my years of therapy and it still affects me. I still have negative reactions to doctors. I'll have to actually talk to Penny about it because she's so puzzled."

Penny does know about her mother's relationship to Munchausen's-by-proxy and to Munchausen's syndrome. When I stayed with Betty in Heritage House a few years ago, Penny and I talked about these conditions at length. Betty believes that her mother got attention by bringing Betty to doctors, claiming she was sick—the classic Munchausen's-by-proxy scenario. But I believe that Betty got sick in order to get her mother's attention, simple Munchausen's, and that she has repeated this pattern in her life. I've talked about my belief with Ellyn, after she became a kabalistic therapist. "Souls strive to be whole in whatever way they can," she tells me. "This is the only way Betty knows to move toward wholeness." And I've told Betty what I believe, but I doubt she really heard what I was saying. What a radical shift in her thinking and behavior would be required if she agreed with me, and acted upon it. And if I'm wrong, what radical shift would be required from me?

Now Betty says, "Laurel, I love you. Thank you for not abandoning me."

"I love you too." I say. And I do.

Sunday, January 15

"I was all packed ready to go to the new hospital room, already on the gurney, and then was told I couldn't go to the new room because it was on an orthopedic ward," Betty says. "So I called the hospital administrator, yelled, and got the room. Still have some fight left in me."

Monday, January 16

Betty's on Xanax and back in her apartment in Penny's house. I refuse to phone there until she has her own phone line. Betty calls me and we talk a bit about how happy we are with the Supreme Court validating Oregon's "doctor-assisted suicide" law. "Maybe Ohio will have one too," I say, and then hear someone on her end picking up the phone. I don't like it.

I am going to Cincinnati tomorrow for an overnight with Susan. We've been friends for twenty-five years. She has been married for nine of them, and I've not yet seen her condo or spent time with her miniature poodle, feral cats, or sweet-faced husband.

"I'm going to help Susan with her book project about hope," I tell Betty.

"I have something to say about that," Betty says. She's enthusiastic. "It may sound like an oxymoron, but hope and terminal illness go together."

This is the first time I've heard Betty say the words "terminal illness."

"I'm happier now than I've ever been in my life," she says. "I'm living for today, and I feel that things are going to be good today. That's how hopefulness and terminal illness overlap."

I don't quite get her reasoning but I like the Laurelism—looking on the bright side.

"My expectations have come way down," she continues. "Who would ever have expected me to be willing and able to live with my child?"

"Another passage," I say. I've been physically altering Gail Sheehy's book *New Passages*. My friend Julie introduced me to altered books, and for the past year I have been fascinated with the process—literally changing books by tearing out pages or smudging them, by drawing or waxing on the page, by highlighting words or adding my own. It's a reclaiming and revisioning process that melds the written and the visual, the old with the new. The sweet scent of beeswax fills the air.

"The things you hope for change as you go through the decades of your life." Betty's on a toot. "Marriage, kids, careers, fame, fortune. . . . Then you hope you live long enough to appreciate it and you hope to die fast, which I haven't seemed to be able to do. . . . I didn't do much with my life, but I raised this amazing child. I did do that."

Friday, January 20

Now that I'm not calling Betty, I have a greater desire to use her idioms, write them, as if doing so will keep our relationship, if not Betty, alive. So to borrow one of Betty's phrases, my overnight with Susan was "quite lovely." We shopped for artist papers, gifts, and charms at St. Theresa's

Textile Trove, Kilimanjaro, One Thousand Villages, and Hyde Park boutiques. For my memoir group friend Bev I bought cocktail napkins featuring a dazed woman in a pink taffeta strapless gown saying, "I was never meant to work." Bev's struggling with the idea of retiring.

Susan and I have always talked easily about our spiritual journeys, as different as they have ostensibly been. Her journey has brought her to Catholicism. Mine has taken me from my mixed Jewish-Protestant background, to nothing, to women's spirituality, to Unitarianism, to Reform Judaism—and here I am searching again.

During my visit Susan and I talked about spirits and reincarnation, prayer and meditation. And we talked about hope, love, and charity—well, not quite the last, although Susan asked about Betty.

"I may be out of line to say this, but you seem to do all the giving," Susan began. "What are you getting from Betty?"

"My memoir writing group asks me the same thing," I reassured Susan that she was not out of line.

What is my need?

"So what do you get?" Susan asked.

"Well, Betty and I have been friends for thirty-five years. She knows my history, loves my children, loves me. She wishes me and mine well in this world. She's family. We've had a deep spiritual connection. If I were to meet her now, no, we wouldn't *become* friends. I pride myself on my loyalty."

"Maybe that's why you've been reincarnated," Susan said, a comment which surprised me.

"Do you think I was disloyal in a previous life and I'm working out my karma?"

"Or you have been too loyal—and you need to learn limits."

On the drive home I was very tired. I listened to a storyteller on NPR's *This American Life.* My eyelids drooped. My tires rumbled. A different storyteller was in the midst of a different story. I must have fallen asleep at the wheel. I opened my window, patted my face, and opened my mouth wide, breathing, forcing myself to stay awake for the last thirty miles. I knew I was foolish not to stop for coffee, but I didn't care. I didn't want to stop. I wanted to get home.

Home, going to sleep, I was so tired I wondered if I was having a heart attack. I had read somewhere that tiredness signals a heart attack in women. I dreamt that I had been applying for grants, working very hard, and then I said to myself, in the dream, *Why are you working? You don't have to work anymore.*

I think about loyalty. To be loyal is to persevere, which is good, but to be loyal also means not letting go, which is not so good. Try as I might, I have not yet let go of my identity as a university professor. Maybe I don't have to.

Tuesday, January 24

I decide to call Betty.

"Do you remember our last phone call?" Betty asks.

"You were full of hope," I say.

"I must have been channeling something," she says derisively. "Now I don't feel at all hopeful."

"Are you taking your Xanax?"

"I don't need it. Half a tablet every couple of days. That's all."

"Maybe you do need more—more often."

"The Xanax slows my breathing down and puts me to sleep."

"That's good."

"I am very sick."

"I'm sorry."

"When I'm in pain, I can't feel hopeful."

"What hurts?

"My knee. Right in the middle."

"Your arthritis acting up?"

"It's not arthritis. It's wake-me-up-screaming pain."

"Sounds like you've torn something."

"What I wanted to tell you is that I've really grabbed onto something," Betty says, as if she was the one who had called me. "All these years I thought Penny was looking for family. Well, I'm not so sure that's true. I think she has just happened upon a throwback way of life when she moved to Delaware. People here live in extended families and social life is doing something for each other."

"Taking caring of you fits right in then," I say.

"This doesn't happen among the people I know," Betty says.

"Now it does."

Wednesday, January 25

Betty is settling in at her daughter's. She has physical therapy and breathing lessons twice a week. This gives her hope. The doctor has increased her meds. Her weight is coming off, but the pain in her spine is "bloodcurdling." There's a cemetery in the back of Penny's property, but nobody knows who's buried there. "The Smiths" live across the street, but nobody knows them. Betty wonders about the graves and the Smiths, and the trailer junk beside another house whose occupants nobody knows either. Mike spends most of his free time spotting deer in his woods behind the house. Penny and Mike cut down trees for firewood for themselves and all of Mike's relatives.

When I write this way about Betty's life, I feel myself creating distance, writing without emotional investment. It is restful.

Saturday, January 28

At last Betty has her own phone line! She's slipped her phone into her pocket while she visits in Penny's kitchen.

"It's Laurel," she tells Penny. "I'll take it back in my apartment."

I can hear Betty's labored breathing as she walks back. Several minutes pass as I chat about the surprisingly beautiful weather in Columbus, interspersed with "Are you okay?" She is coughing.

"There," she says. "Give me a moment to settle in this chair."

This is the first time in months that I have been privy to Betty in motion. I imagine she is wearing her heavy red sweats, heavy wool socks, and red slippers, and that under the sweats her bony arms and legs are purple with vasculitis. Her face is leathered. Her white-haired head is bowed, almost lowing, the way a cow might. This saddens me.

When she has caught her breath and controlled her coughing, she tells me that seventeen primary care physicians have refused to take her as a new Medicare patient. Swollen feet and ankles make her look like a rhinoceros. She is taking a diuretic but can't take too much because "the loss of potassium for someone in my condition" is not good. The ophthalmologist says new glasses won't help her see because she needs cataract surgery. The word *surgery* frightens her.

"How bad are your eyes?" I ask.

"I can't make sense of what's on TV. I can't see stuff on the shelves."

"Can you read?"

"Close up is okay."

"How's your knee?"

"Fine. The chiropractor cleared it up."

I'm asking about her body parts. I realize I am doing what Betty wants her doctors to do.

The visiting nurse is okay. Home-care people are not. They charge too much, want to stay too long, and are terrible drivers. One was older than Betty!

"This morning," she said, "I felt that this was all too hard. That I can't do this anymore." Her breathing becomes labored again. "I'll do *anything* to stay out of cataract surgery," Betty says.

I want to ask if her obsession with finding a new doctor has to do with making new assisted-suicide plans, but I don't.

Sunday, January 29

"Everything in this house is always in motion. No one can sit down," Betty says.

"Maybe that's why you're there," I suggest.

"I am the stillness around which all this circulates."

Monday, January 30

Betty's back in Kent General Hospital—Dover with a 101-degree fever.

"Poor Penny," Betty says. "I got this flu from Penny, who got it from Jack. Penny is so sick."

"How about your legs? I ask.

"The swelling is down. I'm in pain, and I'm on a lot of antibiotics."

"Sorry."

"I met a primary care doctor here who has a solo practice. He said he'd take me as a patient."

Solo practice is important to Betty because she believes such doctors, having no colleagues or staff looking over their shoulders, have greater leeway in how they might practice.

"My oxygen level is bad."

"What is it?" I ask. I partake nearly unconsciously in this co-constructed script quite often. Betty gives a bit of general information, I ask for more.

"Eighty or ninety. Very low."

"Is one hundred perfect?"

"Yes. But no one's perfect!"

We laugh.

"They did a CAT scan of my lungs," she continues.

Pause.

"I think I told you about this before, the nodule in my lung, it was found when I was in Kent, there was just one and now there are two, and the pulmonologist is talking about cancer."

"I thought Dr. Lee said it was a just a pneumonia scar," I say. If Betty has been living with lung cancer, she has kept it a secret.

"The pulmonologist is talking about giving me a PET scan," she continues, ignoring my comment. PET scans are primarily for locating cancers.

"Are you going to do that?" I ask. Last night I went to an end-of-life panel discussion, where I learned that in the last six months of life a person spends as much money on their medical care, on average, as they had the entire rest of their life. I balk at the idea of spending thousands of Medicare dollars for a test that will not extend her life. But what do I know? No wonder Betty likes this pulmonologist.

"The pulmonologist hasn't told me yet if I am having the scan," she says.

"You know, as a patient, you have the right to make decisions for yourself," I say. I learned that at the panel too.

"Doctors don't do sociology and I don't do medicine," she retorts. "What do I know? And I don't want to know."

"Did your bird-in-a-tree lamp come?" I ask. "How does it look?"

"Lovely," she says. "But it will only take a sixty-watt bulb."

I call the hospital early in the morning. Betty will be there another day.

"Poor Penny," she says. "This is not what she bargained for."

"Maybe she did," I say. Penny's works in emergency medicine.

"I'm in terrible pain," Betty says. "I pulled a muscle in my back from coughing."

In the past fifteen years I have had physical therapy for a broken ankle; pulled ankle ligaments; tendonitis of the foot, hands, and elbow; sciatica; plantar fasciitis twice; frozen shoulder, right and left; hip, knee, and back issues. Writing this list I begin feeling sorry for myself. Reading it back to myself, though, I feel how fortunate I've been, how minor my health problems.

"This hospital is so bad," Betty complains.

"Are you in a different hospital?" I ask, confused. "Is this the same hospital you liked yesterday?"

"Same one. I am in so much pain. The doctor ordered a heating pad and it took six hours to get here."

"Where's the pulled muscle?"

"In my back. By my waist."

I try to imagine how coughing could pull a muscle that far down on the back, and I find myself wondering whether Betty has a broken rib or cancer in her bones—or if her spine is fracturing from osteoporosis.

"They can't do a PET scan while I'm in the hospital, it has to be outpatient," she says. "I think I'll go home tomorrow."

"One of the other things I learned from hospice is that if you don't want to go home—" I begin.

"I want to go home. I've been here too long already."

"If you don't want to go home, just tell them you're going to appeal it. *Appeal* is the magic word."

"I want to go home and get the PET scan."

I'm quiet.

"Gives me something to do," she says.

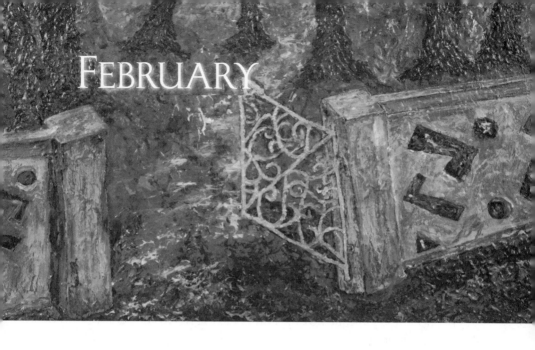

FEBRUARY

Wednesday, February 1

"This horrible hospital," Betty complains. She has an edginess to her voice I haven't heard for a while.

"Penny," she calls out, "Get me a hamburger with onions, and no French fries."

"May I talk to Penny?" I ask.

"Sure. . . . Pen, it's Laurel."

Penny and I talk a bit about this and that, and then I say, "Penny, this might not be the best time to raise this, but if your mom should . . . ah . . . pass over while I am in Australia, would you be willing to have the memorial service after I return?" I have practiced this question for weeks, and I am relieved to have asked it.

"How long will you be in Australia?" Penny asks.

"Six weeks."

Penny talks of this and that and then says, "Good talkin' to you, Laurel."

"You haven't answered my question," I say, surprised at my forthrightness.

"All right, Laurel," says Penny, without much enthusiasm. "Here's Mom again."

"I'll be back soon, Mom," I hear Penny say.

"Poor Penny," Betty says to me.

"How's your pain?" I ask.

"Terrible. The doctor ordered one of those pain patches four hours ago and it's still not here."

"How's your apartment?"

"Everything's topsy-turvy. Mike wants to do everything for me. It ain't gonna work that way. Things haven't found their places yet. Still need a toilet paper holder. My kitchen doesn't have a grater. I'm like my grandma scraping carrots with a knife."

"I like doing that," I say. "I like roughing up the carrot, the coarse texture against my hand, the smell."

The next time someone asks me how come I've stayed friends with Betty, I'll tell them *because both our grandmothers made chicken soup with de-strung celery, peeled onions, and knife-scraped carrots.*

Thursday, February 2

Ten a.m. and Betty's back in her apartment, in pain, waiting for her pain pads. Penny's been waiting at the drugstore for two hours, only to learn that the drugstore doesn't stock them. Mike will try another store while Betty waits for a doctor's phone call.

"I'll catch you later today," I say.

Seven p.m. and my day and dinner finished, I call Betty. "You sound good," I say, responding to her deep pitched "Hello."

"That's the funniest thing I've heard all day," she says.

"What's so funny?"

"I feel awful. I am in so much pain. I've been in bed all day."

"Pulled muscles hurt."

"Penny thinks maybe it's something else. I've been on a muscle relaxant and it hasn't helped at all." Betty starts coughing uncontrollably. "Ouch. *Cough.* Ouch. *Cough.* Ouch!"

Hearing her screams, my eyes tear, the way they did when my children cried in pain.

"Can you take cough suppressants?" Here I am again, trying to fix the problem.

"No," she says angrily. "I'm not supposed to take muscle relaxants either." *Why then has your doctor prescribed them?*

"Every time I cough . . . this is too much . . . ouch . . . the pain is right on my spine."

"Why can't you take muscle relaxants?" *Maybe I'm trying to escape her cries of pain through rational conversation.*

"Oh, what do I know!" she says.

"I am so sorry." *I say this so often. What else is there to say?*

"Penny thinks it's something else, not muscles," Betty says.

"Maybe sciatica," I suggest. *I do not say maybe it's cancer or maybe bones are fracturing when she coughs.*

"Penny thinks it is not good for me to be in my bedroom all day, so she and Mike have turned my apartment upside down. They've brought my hospital bed into the living room so I can watch TV. I sleep in the living room now."

"That's different."

"Penny thinks this pain is not enough to matter. She doesn't understand."

Penny thinks, Penny says, Penny this, Penny that. Is Penny her Mommy?

"How did Penny get her name?" I ask, surprised that I don't know.

"Well, it had to be a P name after my mother."

Why? I wonder. Betty detested her mother.

"What I did to Penny is what my mother did to me," Betty continues. "I gave her a nickname."

Betty didn't quite do what her mother did, though. New Jersey law required that a child be named before it could leave the hospital. "What's your name?" Betty's mother asked the discharge nurse. "Betty," the nurse said. "That'll do," said her mother.

"Well, Ms. Bet, have you figured out how to avoid hospitals forevermore?" *I've wanted to ask her this question for weeks now.*

"I've been studying up on that for years," she says.

"Do you have pills?"

"Yes."

"Doctors can't make people take their pain pills or prevent them from getting more and stashing them," I say, supporting her.

"I need to have this conversation."

"With me?"

"No, not with you. With Penny. . . . Pam's in town and wants to visit," Betty says. "I told her not to."

"Why?"

"I've always told you if I can hold onto my dignity and sense of humor, that's enough. Wearing diapers, lying on a hospital bed in the middle of the living room—it's not funny, and where's the dignity?"

Friday, February 3

"This always happens." Betty sounds annoyed.

"What?"

"You always call when I'm just off the phone."

I'm confused. "You are *off* the phone, aren't you?"

"Nobody calls all day and then everybody calls at once," she says.

"Is Pam coming to see you tomorrow?"

"She's not going to see me."

"Maybe you could put on a nice robe."

"She can't *see* me!" Betty's anger is rising. "I have to let her come out here, though."

"Why?"

"She's bringing things I need from Kent."

"Who's that in my house?" Betty shouts.

I hear a male voice.

"Is that you Jack?" she asks. "Can't you knock?"

"How do you want your sausage cooked?" I hear Jack ask.

"Let Mike surprise me."

"How do you want it cooked?" Jack repeats. He must have orders to get Grandma's order right.

"Surprise me," she repeats.

"I thought you'd have eaten by now," I say. It's 7:30.

"Yeah, that's what I would have thought. Can I call you back later?"

"Sure. Whenever."

The evening passes and Betty does not call back. Ernest and I watch *Survivor* and *Without a Trace* on our TiVo, and I straighten up my desk yet again. I am totally exhausted even though I have napped twice today. I look at my list of things to do before I go to Australia. On the list is sending my essay "Jeopardy" to *Qualitative Inquiry*. I spend a few minutes writing an abstract, cover letter, and title page. "Jeopardy" has been in my file cabinet for eight years.

Saturday, February 4

I reread "Jeopardy." It chronicles the marriage of my son Josh to Rachel, the birth of their son, Akiva, and the breakup of their marriage. Rachel was forty-three at the time of the pregnancy, no medical tests, interventions, preventions, doctors, or hospitals were involved in the birthing or aftercare of Akiva. As his tie-dyed baby shirt attested, he was "Born at Home by CHOICE." He had a tied tongue that the midwife cut with a knife. He was jaundiced and was placed on a sunny windowsill. His umbilical cord was put in the freezer to be buried in the spring.

Rachel believes in birth and death as "spiritual gateways." The newborn, like the dying one, is fragile during the passage, susceptible to destructive energies. For Akiva's first three months, she limits my visits. I worry that he will catch a terrible disease or never talk right or that he is genetically damaged. Rachel doesn't believe in any vaccinations, including polio. At four months Akiva contracts whooping cough. At six months he's exposed to a child who was given the live polio vaccine. I do not have the heart to fully love a grandchild I might lose. Only when his first birthday passes and he is still alive, walking, and talking, do I relax my fears.

It is very painful for me to revisit that time.

I thought I had buried this paper in my files because it was not flattering to Rachel. But as I reread it, I see it is not flattering to me either. I appear inadequate in the face of life, and in the face of death.

Why did I choose to reread "Jeopardy?" I have a long list of things that must get done. But maybe what's not on the list is the most important: learning about my long-term relationship to fragility and death. I see a shadow of myself, in a glass, darkly.

I want to talk to Betty about all of this. But I cannot. *That* Betty— the friend who knows my family's history—is not up to the conversation

I want to have. I put "Jeopardy" back in the file cabinet. I am not ready to expose myself to the whole world, and the whole world or even a tiny part of it just won't give a damn, won't care the way my friend Betty has.

Every time I think I have worked through Betty's death and dying, I am wrong. How intense my sorrow is. In five days I leave for my six-week sojourn in Australia and Tahiti. While I am away, will my friend have gone through the spiritual gateway?

I return to my list of things to do. I call my older brother, Barrie, in Shreveport. He's been kneading bread and thinking about mother and me. Yesterday he went to the grocery store and bought food he doesn't usually buy—cottage cheese, sour cream, salami. Food from our childhood.

"Do you like baked sweet potatoes?" Barrie asks.

"I love them," I say. "I hate coconut."

"I can't stand coconut either," he says. "Our tastes come from our heritage; they're learned."

"I think it's partly genetic," I say.

I don't tell him that I have been writing about mothering, learned behavior, and genetics, and that I think we've been communicating through whatever spiritual gateway siblings might share.

"I was not a good son. I wasn't interested in Father's stories."

"I didn't ask him either," I say. I'm an interviewer. I ask other people about their lives, but I asked my father little about his. Most of what I know about his early life comes through hearsay.

"I wasn't a good brother either," Barrie continues.

When we were young he threatened, teased, and tormented me. It's a wonder I lived through the "tests" he gave me, like cutting me in half for his magic show. When we were teenagers, though, he was an excellent big brother, protecting me from the "bad guys" and fixing me up with the "good guys." Now we're friends.

"My friend Betty will probably die while I'm gone," I say.

"That's probably a good way to say good-bye."

"I don't think so—"

"Whoops! There goes the bell signaling my bread has risen! Have a great trip."

Snowy and windy and eighteen degrees last night. All my joints are unhappy. Today is the day Ernest and I take Mimi-the-cat to my friend Pat's house in the country. We pack Mimi's Scoop litter, Aquari-Yums, Iams Adult Diet, organic catnip, and the pink blanket that she sleeps on when she sleeps on my bed. It is a forty-five-minute drive. She does better than expected in the car, mi-mi-ing just a bit now and then. At Pat's she jumps out of her carrying case, sniffs Tipper, who sniffs her back, and then Mimi sniffs out the other three cats who live there. Not a hiss or a howl do we hear. When we leave, all five cats are curled like littermates in the basement behind a cardboard shield. Mimi likes it here. She is on vacation.

Our home seems empty without Mimi yowling for treats. I do my e-mail and call a couple of friends to say good-bye. Then I call Betty. Her voice is raspy, worse than usual. Her coughing is labored, almost like choking, sounding the way Mimi sounds when she's trying to expel a hairball.

"How're you?" I ask.

"I've felt better," she says.

"How was Pam's visit?"

"Humiliating. Her husband came too, and her niece."

"And you don't even know her." I'm imagining how embarrassed I would feel.

"They had the good sense to cut the visit short," she says.

"So what did Pam bring?"

"My CDs and my wicker bed tray."

And pills?

"This can't go on," Betty says. "I'm in too much pain. I just don't know who I am. It changes so fast. I'm not the person I was. I'm not even the person I was a month ago when I came here to Penny's."

"Is Penny there now?"

"No."

"What about Mike?"

"Penny's at the beach with Jack, watching the Polar Bear Club. And Mike's playing poker at the firehouse."

"So . . . you're alone?"

"Yes. All I can do is lie here and watch football until Penny comes home."

Why did they leave her alone if she's in as bad straits as she says she is? I decide to keep her on the phone until Penny returns.

"Speaking of sports, I have something to say!"

"You? Sports? That's a joke," Betty says.

If Betty's phone ever rings during the last crucial minutes of a live-televised sports event, she knows it's me because "everyone else in the world is watching the game."

"Columbus has a pro hockey team now," I say.

"Er, Laurel. Yes. The Blue Jackets."

"Oh, so you know about them too?" I am stalling for time, trying to keep Betty entertained. "Anyway, the Arena District taverns are strictly enforcing a new rule that prohibits patrons from wearing a T-shirt or cap of any team that is not playing that day in the arena."

"Yeah, and?"

"I don't get it," I conclude.

"Neither do I," she says. "But it's not as bad as having people expelled from the House gallery for wearing political T-shirts. Tsk-tsk, democracy is dead in America. In the House of Representatives, for God's sake, no free speech."

"The House makes its own rules," I say.

"So what?"

"So it's not about free speech—it's about decorum. They probably had these rules in 1777. No politicking in the gallery."

"The House. That's what I mean," Betty says. "No free speech in the House anymore."

"What do you mean *anymore*? Women were expelled during the fight to pass the Equal Rights Amendment."

"Ah, yes. Betty Friedan. Her death has hit me hard," Betty says. "I so disliked her as a person but loved what she did for my life."

"Why didn't you like her?"

"Instead of being gracious when famous, she became . . . *cough cough* ouch! . . ."

"Abrasive?" I fill in the word. As Betty coughs, I continue, "Betty Friedan wanted her gravestone to say that she helped women feel better about themselves so they could more freely and fully love men."

"Sounds like her!" Betty scoffs. "Who'd want to love the stupid men running things now? Tsk-tsk. No free speech in the House anymore."

"We've never been allowed to distribute leaflets close to polling places either," I say, trying to keep Betty on the phone. "Does that abrogate free speech?"

"Talking politics with you is scary," she says.

"Why?"

"Because we disagree."

"You're very passionate and committed," I say. "I'm more analytical. We've been on different political paths for a long time. Ever since you thought that O. J. was innocent."

"Even before that," she says.

"And we're still friends," I say.

"This sounds like a good place to stop."

"Well . . . um . . . ah . . ."

"And here's Penny."

When we hang up, I realize that this is the longest, most wide-ranging, most potentially conflictual conversation we've had in years. Do I sense that there will not be any of these in the future?

Before dinner I notice that the Thanksgiving turkey's wishbone is still drying on the kitchen windowsill. A poem I wrote years ago comes to me:

> You take one end
> I the other
> Pulling each
> Against each
> Until the bone
> Breaks

Monday, February 6

When I described Betty's complaint of sharp back pain to my physical therapist this morning, he said, "sounds like Valsalva. It's like squeezing a fire hose." That made no sense to me, so when I go home I download ten pages from several different websites. My tendency to catastrophize when I feel powerless is diminished by getting a little knowledge.

The Valsalva mechanism, I learn, coordinates muscles so that air pressure in the lungs will automatically close the upper airway. But when someone with compromised lungs and a languishing body coughs, the stress on the abdomen can strain the back muscles, leading to fractured bones in the back. Another stage in Betty's COPD. I delete the downloads.

After lunch I go to my new hairdresser, who colors me blondish, cuts me short, and lo! My hair is no longer dragged down and straight but curly. I think fondly of the time when I dyed Betty's hair. The kids and grandkids come for supper, and afterward I return to my packing. Nothing quite gets done, nothing is checked off my list.

I'm about to try on my travel pants to see if they still fit, when the phone rings.

"Stay calm under all circumstances," Betty says. Her voice sounds stronger.

I tell her about my busy day.

"Opals," she says. "There are opals in Australia." The opal is Betty's birthstone. "Get yourself something beautiful with an opal in it."

"I'll claim it's an early birthday gift from you to me," I say. I'd read somewhere that it's bad luck to give yourself an opal.

"You're going to Tahiti on your way back, right?"

"Yes!" I am thrilled about this exotic trip.

"Pearls," she says. "There are black pearls in Tahiti. Get yourself something beautiful with a pearl in it."

"Shall I look in the womb of a black-lipped mollusk?" I ask. I've been reading about black pearls. I'm showing off.

"Beware the black-lip mother of pearl doesn't give you a black eye with its ink." Betty has not been reading about black pearls. She's not showing off either. She knows a lot of trivia.

"How's your reading going?" I ask.

"The ophthalmologist says do the cataract surgery, but I'm ignoring him."

"How's the new aide?" I ask.

"She's good. I spent most of the morning getting a shower. Tomorrow I'm going to wash my hair."

Betty says "I" when in fact it's a "she" who showers her, washes her hair, changes her bedclothes.

"Do you have your wheelchair?"

"And a walker. And I walked five steps today without it."

"Great improvement," I say. "Are you going to get the PET scan?"

"What's the point? Only that it will give me something to do for a day. But I couldn't do it physically anyway . . . couldn't lie on my back in the hard scanner. I have calls in now for all my doctors."

That'll give you something to do.

"Do you want to hear your horoscope for today? It's probably different from the one in your paper."

"Ha! I can't read newsprint, Laurel," she says.

"Well, here's your horoscope: 'It is said that you can never go back. What it really means is that when you go back, it's not the same, so you're not really back. Nonetheless, today you get as close to *back* as possible without being there.'"

"I shed a tear about Betty Friedan today," Betty says. "And I was brought back to the spring-summer of 1970, the most momentous three months in my life. The shootings at Kent State, my father got remarried, I went to Washington for the sociology meetings, and I saw Al for the first time in years, and I met you. I took the train from Newark to Washington—read *The Feminine Mystique*—and when I got off the train I was a different person. My life was never the same. The first sign I saw at the meetings was one that said 'Woman's Caucus.' I can't go back. But there I am."

Tuesday, February 7

Of late, to start the day with some fun I have been casually testing my bridgemanship by figuring out the bids and plays in the *Dispatch*'s daily bridge column. I'm still pretty good at it. For today's column I played in my mind the one-club convention and made good on my heart doubleton.

When I was seven I became the fourth for bridge in my house. My older sister, Jessica, taught me the Goren bidding method for counting card points. When play began, I became the dummy. Partnerless, sitting out the hand, I walked about, looked at everyone's cards, and followed the play. In college a friend, later to be a Life Bridge Master, taught me the subtleties of contract bridge. Our partnership made us money. Much later I discovered duplicate bridge, in which, because the same hand is played by different players, luck is eliminated. The first time I played, I won the tournament. I've not played for thirty years, though, because when I play, I become a narrow, competitive, critical, demanding, uncompromising, self-absorbed, show-offy soul. It's not *me* playing—it's my shadow self.

I decide to call my sister in Des Moines.

"How's John?" I ask. Jessica's husband, John, has been part of my life since I was seven. He taught me algebra, chemistry, and bike riding, and gave me dimes to leave him alone in the living room with my sister, both then high school sophomores. Instead, I'd hide behind Father's red leather chair. Sometimes I was John's bridge bidding partner. When he was a Marine in Korea, his sisters, thinking he had been killed, sold all his belongings. Now he has congestive heart failure.

"We're good here," Jessica says. "John's at infusion."

We chat for close to an hour, a luxury I have been giving myself of late, since Betty's pronounced illness.

"Are you all packed?" Jessica attends to the needs and details of my life.

"Guess I'd better do that."

"Love ya a bunch," she says.

After I'm packed, I shop for Valentine's Day cards. There are cards for women friends to send one another. "I got you something for Valentine's Day," says one. Inside there's a grungy, beer-guzzling, unshaven, unkempt guy. "He's expecting your call," says the tag line. In another, two elderly women are talking about sex. "Do I look like I've never done it?" one asks, appraising herself in the mirror on her diamond-studded compact. "Friends don't let friends be alone on Valentine's Day," says another card. The inside is rated XXX.

The friend cards assume both friends are single and seeking, if not the love and partnership of a man, at least a sexual encounter, no matter how gross. The idea that two women could be best friends and want to acknowledge their partnership is not marketable, or marketed.

I suppress the reborn temptation of the bridge decks, two to a box.

I choose a loving (and sexy) card for my Ernest, and browse the pop-up cards, choosing one for Betty. When opened, a wordless peacock pops out, tail feathers unfurled, each feather tipped with a little glittery heart. His head bobbles. He reigns over a bed of flowers. So many times Betty and I met at Kingswood Gardens and nodded our heads in gleeful approval over the peacocks and peahens, free-ranging over crowds of daffodils.

Wednesday, February 8

Time to send my last e-mails before I turn off my computer. I send one to Betty's friend Ellyn, the only person in Betty's world with whom I can be completely honest.

Date: Wed. 08, Feb 2006
From: richardson
To: eg336
Subject: Re: I'm going to Australia

hi ellyn—i'm going to Australia tomorrow for six weeks!!! Returning via Tahiti!! (i've attached my itinerary). i'll be able to get e-mail (after about a week). doing writing workshops at various universities. . . . ernest is coming too—it's a freebie for him. . . . I don't know if Betty will still be with us when i get back—she is weak, as you know, and dispirited one moment and happy the next (i think that's when the Xanax kicks in). . . . anyway, i wanted to touch base with you (or flirt in the ether waves). . . . not always easy for Penny to communicate—but I know you'll let me know if I need to know something. . . . cheers and happy valentine's day,

laurel

Was it mere forgetfulness on my part? When I discover that I don't have Betty's new Delaware phone number in my travel address book, the airplane's already taxiing toward the runway with Ernest's and my three duffle bags, two carry-ons, two sleep apnea machines, and us heading to Los Angeles, where we will board Qantas to Australia, to arrive in Hobart, Tasmania, twenty-two hours after our departure.

After my father's death, I became afraid of flying, but my fear didn't totally ground me. I'd take a bite of Valium and fall asleep. Lately my fear has vanished, maybe because I've lived through plane problems, proving that pilots know what they're doing. Maybe because I am older and feel I've lived a full life. But I still get flight jitters, free-floating anxiety, and am a bit obsessive about wanting everything in its rightful place.

Not having Betty's number has jangled my nerves. I call Penny on my cell phone. I'm grateful she's home—she often isn't—and grateful she answers the phone. Like everyone else in her generation, it seems, she often doesn't. "I'm on the plane going to Australia," I tell her, "and I don't have Betty's new phone number."

"Yeah," she says. "It's hard to find it."

I don't think she's listening to what I said.

"Take your shoes off now," I overhear her say to Jack. He's grousing in the background.

Poor Penny: big-time work crises, caretaker of a son and a mother, and now here I come with my mini-crisis.

"I guess you're busy," I say, "but can you give me Betty's phone number?"

"Just wait a minute," I hear her say.

"I really can't wait," I say, more harshly than I intended. "The plane is taxiing."

"No. Not you, Laurel. I was telling Jack to wait. Here's Mom's number."

I thank her and call Betty.

"How's your breathing?" I ask. My breathing is fast and shallow.

"It comes and goes."

I laugh at the little joke, but Betty doesn't.

"I've been living my life around your leaving and now you've left," she says. "I can't get my mind around it."

I can't get my mind around what she's saying.

"Turn off all electronic devices, cell phones, and laptops," the flight attendant intones over the PA system.

"Talk to you later," I say.

"Take notes about everything," Betty says. "Write about it."

We arrive at 8 p.m. at Los Angeles LAX. What a rude, obnoxious, noisy spot of concrete. Getting ourselves from the domestic to the international terminal in the smog, congestion, and ear-piercing whistles and horns was a nightmare. Had we spent the night here, as our travel agent suggested, we'd have had our luggage to lug around too. So this is what has happened to "my" pleasant airport—the one I knew when I lived in southern California forty years ago.

Our Qantas Boeing 767 flight takes off on time, at 11 p.m. Each seat has an individual video screen, and each passenger can choose private entertainment from an extensive list of movies, music, television reruns. Attendants pass out snack packs, bottled Fiji water, and goody bags containing earphones, earplugs, socks, eye mask, tooth-cleaning stuff, and a deck of miniature cards. The lights are turned off, and silence prevails for the next twelve hours. I sleep and awaken a day later, having crossed the international date line, to the smell of coffee and omelets. I like Qantas.

The Tasmania airport in Hobart is blissfully quiet. No cells ringing, no one shouting into the air, no one's private business made public, no groups of rowdy teenagers, no televisions, no confused groups of tourists. We exchange American dollars for Australian ones and I buy a twenty-dollar phone card. It'll cost me 3.4 cents per minute to phone America plus a 60-cent "call-up" charge. Plus figuring out when someone in America will be available at the same time that I am. There is a sixteen-hour and one-day time difference, forward or backward, I don't know which.

Ernest drives our mini-Nissan on the "wrong side" of the road to the Hotel Mercuré. Betty and I have a standing joke about me and hotels. If Betty arrives first, she never unpacks because she knows I'll be bitching about the room and we'll be moving to another one. I want to call her and complain not just about our room but about the hotel.

Hotel Mercuré is a square limestone affair on the edge of a commercial district, not charming or on the water, as I had supposed it would be. When we open the window to let the smoke out, the traffic noise comes in. We walk the mile into town through sex shops, tattoo parlors, and warehouses. Ernest's legs are swollen from the flight. We're tired. I'm thinking, *Betty, aren't you glad you're not here listening to my whining?*

But all is not lost! Hotel Mercuré's food is surprisingly good. Its closet-sized gift shop contains lovely local crafts, where I buy a beautiful opal-studded wooden bookmark as a gift to myself from Betty. The traffic noise does settle down, and Hobart is bathed in clean air and silence. Then comes white rain, heavy rain, translucent, with the sun shining through it. We're almost to Antarctica, and the winds off the sea are bracing. When the rain and the winds subside, the light feels magical.

Tasmania's slogan is Expect the Unexpected.

Sunday, February 12

"I think it would be really hard to leave this place," I say to a middle-aged petrol station clerk at a junction on the River Runs Trail.

"Dunno," the woman says. "Never have."

I envy her and all the others in this world who know their place. Betty has come to know Kent, Ohio, as "her place" by living there, and living through her distaste for the midwestern landscape, the lake-effect snow, and the "goyishness" of the people until she arrived at the place where she has friends, political allies, and a deep affection for daffodils. She wants to live long enough to go home to Kent to die.

Ten years ago Sedona was her place, but because of her struggles to breathe in the rarified air, her total dependence on the goodwill of strangers, and her feeling that she'd exhausted the spiritual gifts of the area, Sedona could no longer be her place. She has asked me to scatter some of her ashes there, though.

For most of my adult life I have searched for a place, "my place." I've lived in Ohio for forty-two years, but it's still not my place. I've been to forty-nine of the states, lived in San Francisco, New York City, Seattle, and Boulder. I've traveled through Europe, Mexico, Canada, Lebanon, Israel, Iceland, Russia, and now Tasmania. Only Chicago, where I was born and raised, and Sedona, where I feel at peace, have ever felt like they might be my place. But I can't imagine constructing a life in either of them. As I write this, I am thinking about my study at home, my spring green walls and forest green swivel chair, my picture window framing our lush backyard, in summer as green as the famous green of Ireland. I am always comfortable in my study space. Maybe if I mentally downsize place to space, I will stop moaning, like a heartsick romantic, for something that may not exist. Betty is the romantic, but I think she has come to understand, as I have not, that a place does not magically appear, like Brigadoon. You make your place.

When Betty asked me why I wanted to go to Tasmania so much, I told her so I could say, "I've been there," and to see a genuine Tasmanian devil and the Penal Colony ruins at Port Arthur. I didn't tell her, to find out if it was my place.

Ernest drives us on the Convict Trail to Port Arthur's penal colony. The roads are bermless, the towns simple and cared for, the landscape open with rocky outcroppings—or are those sheep? Yes, hundreds of free-ranging sheared sheep.

We pay our entrance fee, accept our prisoner identity cards, and eat a snack at Felon's Restaurant. Neither of us wants to spend time in the museum. We want to explore the ruins. The suffering of those imprisoned here, many mere children, seems present in the crumbling walls of the closet-sized cells. The prison gloss, that many convicts learned useful skills, does not override our grief. Neither of us wants souvenirs.

We take the little boat to the Isle of the Dead, a small island in the bay. Prisoners decompose in mass unmarked graves down the hill. Guards and administrators are preserved in marked graves up the hill. The highest ranked are commemorated with grotesquely large gravestones and fancifully wrought iron fences at the very top of the hill. Beneath one downhill slope the convict children decompose, and little

Tasmanian oak trees have sprung from their bones. A little boy hides behind a sapling. Ernest takes his picture. I place a stone by the sapling to honor the buried child. We are very moved by this little island, and on our drive back to Hobart we discuss how and where we might be buried. Betty's way ahead of me on this one.

Monday, February 13

"Do you want to pet Patsy?" Jack-the-keeper asks us. Patsy is a six-month-old wombat whose mother was killed by a car. Ernest and I have driven to Something Wild, a sanctuary for displaced and injured animals.

"Do I ever!" I say.

The baby wombat is adorable. That is the perfect word to describe her. She is the size of a six-month-old human baby. She looks at us with open, warm-watery eyes, totally trusting. Her fur is soft and plushy. Her nose is velvety wet. At eighteen months, Jack-the-keeper tells us, she'll viciously turn on her human caretakers. They'll put her in a blind with food and water near where she came from and help her reacclimate herself to her own world, burrowed for most of her future life deep in the ground, emerging only now and then for food and sex. Patsy will definitely know her place.

"Do you want to see the devils?" Jack asks.

Enclosed in a space smaller than my backyard are a Tasmanian devil "couple" and their four newly weaned offspring. This is the first couple that didn't kill each other while being mated in captivity, thanks to the dissertation research efforts of a woman who discovered exactly when the female devil would be receptive to the male. I didn't ask *how* she discovered it but I imagined a tiny thermometer delicately placed. The babies are cute and agile, scavenging inside hollow logs for insects, chasing rodents down, chomping on carrion half hidden under rocks. Their mother's ears turn a bright red to scare us away.

Ernest says, "Wallabies, kangaroo, possums, devils—"

"No koalas, though," I say. Koalas are Betty's favorite animal.

"That's Peter," Jack-the-keeper says, petting a wallaby that has stopped to visit with us. "Peter's one of our animals that just plain refuses to leave the refuge. We take him to a blind, leave him there, and in a couple of days he's back again."

"He thinks he's found his home," I say.

"Come see the platypus. They live here permanently."

We follow our noses to the eucalyptus trees that shade the riverbank and breathe in the complexly sweet aroma. We spot a family of platypus in the river.

"Look how small they are!" I say. "When I learned about them in the *Weekly Reader* in third grade, I thought they were the size of crocodiles."

"But they're near small enough to fit into my shoe," Ernest says. He is limping.

"Wom-bat! Wom-bat!"

Three Japanese teenagers have gathered around Jack, who is feeding Patsy with a little bottle of opossum milk.

"Wom-bat! Wom-bat!" The girls are laughing and shouting.

I take their picture. Each makes the sign of the V. For victory? For peace?

"Wombats are Pokemons!" Ernest says. "Patsy looks like Pichachu!" Ernest has an uncanny ability to recognize faces.

"You're right," I say. Then I realize that we are much farther from our home than these girls are from theirs. I am halfway around the world.

"I can't walk anymore," Ernest says. His double-level BiPAP sleep apnea machine's transformer burned out last night, frying the machine. Without the machine, his severe sleep apnea puts him at risk for a heart attack. He is exhausted. His legs and feet are swollen to twice their normal size, and a nail-sharp pain drives into his left heel whenever he sets his foot down. I think he has plantar fasciitis. We drive to a national park, breathe the eucalyptus-scented air, grateful that our lungs are working, talk to the Tasmanian tiger damsel dragonfly stowed away under our windshield wiper, and drive her and us to Hobart, singing, "Merrily we sing along."

Betty loved driving to out-of-the-way places, heading off on side roads, stopping in cafés in small towns just to see who and what was there. In Arizona we once drove eighty miles out of our way on a gravel road because the map said the road led to a town named Chillin.

Chillin no longer existed, but a Texaco station served fountain Coke and "Famous Chicken-in-the Basket." Betty would get a "hoot," to use her word, out of Tasmania's fast-food chicken restaurants: Chicken Poo, Canadian Chickie, Charcoal Chickie-Chickie, Legs and Breasts, Chicken Feed.

Tuesday, February 14

"Happy Valentine's Day," I say to Ernest, as I give him his card.

"You too," he says, giving me mine.

It's so nice to have simple rituals that are doable no matter where we are.

"Can you walk today?" I ask. Last night I gave him my own sleep apnea machine, and although it is not set to his specifications, I think it helped. My sleep problem is allergy-based, so I sleep well here in Tasmania, where the air is clear.

"I'll be okay," he says. "I slept better."

We're going to the Air Walk over the oldest pine forest in the world. We ride a golf cart to the stairwell. Up we go on the metal risers, high above acres of tree tip-tops, to a 100-foot cantilevered section that is moving up and down, back and forth in the torturous winds. A few intrepid travelers venture out. Ernest is one and I am too. I have vertigo, nausea, awe. Ernest can barely walk. Betty could not have walked this at all. Half a world away, I am here.

On our way back to Hobart, we stop at the corner of Jew Lane and Race Street for lunch at a convict-built stone house, one of many such houses in the charming little town of Greeve. I eat my Australian specialty, breaded and deep-fried lamb chops, and then ask the waitress about the street names. She doesn't know about Race Street, but "once there was a Jew who lived up Jew Lane."

"Lavender will be a nice antidote," I say to Ernest after lunch. "Tower Hill is only a bit out of the way. And there won't be much walking."

Five thousand different kinds of lavender greet us, as does their owner, a woman who took a midlife career change, bought the land, planted the flowers, had a still built from a farmer friend's hand-me-down milking tins, won a best-of-show award in 2004 for her lavender oils, created lavender fudges, and designed lavender-filled bookmarks, eight of which I buy for my memoir writing group. Ernest and I pat our foreheads and wrists with lavender oil. I don't think of grief, illness, or problems back home. Half a world away and a lavender orgy. Is that what it takes?

That night I am so homesick I want to cry.

Thursday, February 16

"No one wants to terrorize Tasmania," I say to Ernest as the security guard waves us through the Tasmania airport checkpoint without checking our passports or carry-ons.

Maisie Lansford, the professor who secured my fellowship, meets us at the Melbourne airport. She is tanned and her hair is a jumble of dark curls. She looks young enough to be my daughter. We give each other big hugs. She admires my Dansko sandals, and I admire her bronze-colored silk jacket. Ernest is quite fatigued, and I am glad there are three of us to cart our luggage to the four-door Commodore Holden that Maisie has borrowed from the University of Melbourne's fleet.

"Good thing my mother taught me to look both ways before crossing the street," I say to Maisie. I am a left-hander who was made a right-hander. The only way I can tell left from right is to say to myself, *You write with your right,* while simultaneously air-writing with my right index finger. The placement, speed, and number of cars is more wrenching, scary, and disorienting for me, I think, than for those who are fortunate enough to have brain and handedness in sync.

Every approaching car startles me, so I am greatly relieved when we reach our destination, the small residential University College. Our apartment is on the second floor at the college's periphery. From the apartment's hallway entrance (the key and doorknob turn backward), I can peer into the bathroom and see its shower, tank toilet, and little pedestal sink (yes, the water drains clockwise). Down our apartment's hallway to the right is a galley kitchen and spacious living room, and to the left is a large bedroom with mirrored folding closet doors. How 1960s!

Outsized windows abut outsized windows in the west-facing

corners of both rooms. Light switches are "hidden" on the door frames, and they switch on-off upside down. The apartment is not air-conditioned and there is a peculiar semisweet odor that we cannot identify.

We'll be "serviced" once a week, and we'll eat three meals a day, if we choose, with staff, other visiting scholars, and the 175 resident undergraduates, a fourth of whom are Asian. Two nights a week we're invited to High Table if we don the academic gowns now stowed in plastic dry-cleaning bags in our closet. Maisie leaves us to unpack.

I finally figure out that morning today in Melbourne is afternoon yesterday in America. I decide to call Betty. After four "please-help-me" phone calls to Reception, I figure out how to call America. This is how:

Pick up phone.

Wait thirty seconds for tone.

Press ##.

Wait thirty seconds—silence.

Press 7962#.

Wait forty seconds for tone.

Press 0.

Wait fifty seconds for tone.

Press 1-300-302-0507—the "800" number for my phone card.

Listen to menu.

"If English, press one."

Press 1.

"Enter code."

Press code numbers.

"You have twenty dollars in your account. Dial your number, country code first."

Press 1-302-Betty's number.

Ring. Ring. Ring.

Pick up, pick up, Betty in America!

"Hi, Betty! We're in Melbourne," I say, flushed with my transoceanic phone success.

"You sound like you're just around the corner," Betty says.

"Yeah. Our connection's better than it is in the states." I tell her about Tasmania's landscapes, plants, and animals. "So how are *you*?" I ask.

"Coughing a lot, as you can hear. My bed's still in the living room. Mike's going to get me a reclining chair so I can have a little more dignity. *Cough. Cough.* I'll see the chiropractor next week. *Cough.* It's very hard. *Cough cough.*"

I think I hear her ribs rattling across her lungs.

"Talk to you later," I say.

"You bet."

Friday, February 17

We settle Ernest into his studio at the Student Union and me into my office in Dean Kingsley's suite. Melbourne, I discover, is a city of seven million and not the charming English town that I had imagined. The University of Melbourne is not an Australian replica of Oxford or Cambridge but a complex of colleges covering vast acreage and serving a student population of forty-five thousand, most of them commuters. The University of Melbourne seems more like the Ohio State University that I left behind than the academia of my dreams.

Saturday, February 18

Saturday morning Maisie drives us and her mother, "Mum," a gray-haired Maisie, in her tiny Holden Barina to Queen Victoria Market, the largest open-air market in the Western Hemisphere, an expanse of exotica—kangaroo fillets, snails, persimmons, flathead fish, lollyshops (candy stores) , long blacks (coffee), oysters, aftermarket computers, devil-red flowers, orange pacifiers, purple panties. There are live yellow chicks—for eating.

I admire Maisie's blue silk mandarin-style jacket.

"It's Vietnamese," she says. "And I'll take you to the booth."

Ernest takes a seat in the booth while I try on jackets.

"I'll buy it for you," Ernest says, admiring me in a black and red satin jacket whose sleeves reach past my fingertips.

He hands the clerk thirty Australian dollars—twenty-three dollars American. Ernest's buying clothing or jewelry for me is a little shopping game we have when we travel. We act as if we are an old-fashioned married couple—she struts, he pays.

"I like it on you," Maisie says.

"Luv-ly," says Mum, holding a crocheted shopping bag full of "veggies."

When you try on clothes and ask your shopping companion how you look, you're allowing yourself to be vulnerable and trusting. Publicly shopping for clothes with a friend is a site of intimacy. I'm picky about my shopping companions.

Betty and I bonded through shopping. Often she and I bought the same outfit in different sizes or colors. "It doesn't matter," we said. "We live in different cities." But I think it did matter. Putting on those clothes was both a symbolic and material way of being *reclothed* in the shared experience, and a way of reconfirming shared tastes and values. I would say, "I'm going to wear the black Carole Little outfit tomorrow." And Betty would say, "I think I'll wear mine too. Good idea." We'd laugh. Years later Betty might say, "I found the Carole Little outfit at the back of my closet. Do you remember it?" And I would say, "Of course. Does it still fit you? Mine has been long gone too small." And then we'd talk about our how our bodies have changed and reminisce about our lives when we bought those Carole Little outfits at Saks in Washington, D.C., gleefully escaping from that year's sociology convention.

It has been seven years now since Betty and I have gone clothes shopping together, another one of our losses. As I put on my Vietnamese jacket, I wonder if Maisie and I will be shopping friends.

Sunday, February 19

On Sunday Ernest and I walk five minutes to the tram stop, take it to Federation Square, admire the postmodern architecture, ooh over the Aboriginal art in the museum, walk to the Arts Centre: a mega-urban space alongside the river, in whose black box I am to do a workshop— "Telling Lives"—for visual artists, writers, and circus performers. *My God, this is big! And it's downtown! Yikes!*

I have preperformance jitters.

We walk back to the square. Ernest's heel is hurting, and he is relieved to find a vacant table at the outdoor café. We experience food sticker shock—a couple of sandwiches and two Diet Cokes coming in at seventy dollars Australian. We relax into the Australian jazz trio playing classic American jazz under the orange and turquoise awnings of the square on a sunny afternoon. When we get home I call Betty, but she is coughing too much to talk.

I am having more and more trouble breathing too. I cough as soon as I enter the apartment. Its smell is becoming more acrid. My nose is running. I am taking a nightly sleeping pill, getting more and more tired.

Monday, February 20

Monday morning Ernest and I walk the five minutes from our apartment to the dining room for an eight o'clock breakfast. Available are white toast, cinnamon bread toast, English muffins, peanut butter and jelly, Vegamite, Weetamix, milk, orange juice, coffee, and tea. Only on Tuesdays and Thursdays is there "hot breakfast." I pick up my "take-away" lunch: a tuna sandwich, apple, and boxed juice. Ernest picks up his: two chicken-loaf sandwiches, apple, and boxed juice. We walk the five minutes back to our apartment. I try calling Betty. No answer. Maybe she's at the doctor's.

At nine o'clock Ernest and I begin our walk to his studio and my office. We walk the five minutes to the tram stop, cross two heavily trafficked streets, walk a quarter mile, enter the university through the gates of Trinity College, note the depleted cases of champagne, detritus of the students' al fresco breakfast, walk past the cricket and sports centre, turn up Tin Alley, step on chalked announcements—"Free Beer, This Way"—follow the arrows to the Student Union, walk through hordes of students gathered around the free beer, enter the building, ride the lift to Ernest's third-floor studio. A room of his own, with windows from floor to ceiling. We have been walking for twenty-five minutes.

I kiss Ernest good-bye and begin the second leg of my journey. I walk past hordes of beer-besotted students; walk on the Christian Union ads, chalked in English and Chinese; walk to the post office, where I get kangaroo postcards; cut through the architecture and social science buildings to Alice Hoy; and up the flight of stairs to my office in Dean Kingsley's suite. Another fifteen minutes have passed. The temperature is in the eighties. I am tired and hot. Blessedly, my office is air-conditioned. The faculty offices are not.

Eleven days have passed since I last logged onto my e-mail. Four hundred twenty-six "Not Spam" messages await me, including an e-mail from Pat, regarding Mimi-the-cat. "She's doing fine," Pat writes. "She's become best friends with Boots. Don't worry about her, and enjoy your trip." Betty's friend Ellyn has e-mailed too:

Date: Thursday, 09, Feb 2006
To: richardson
From: eg336
Subject: re: I'm going to Australia
Oh Sweetie,

My denial system is so apt. I think Betty will continue in this up/down mode indefinitely.

I call a few times a week. It's hard to listen to her breathe.

The Xanax "should" take the edge off her anxiety. God knows what the interactions of all the drugs are. I'm glad she's in Delaware because she seems to be glad. Although in Kent she has more in-house company/services.

Anyhow, enjoy "down under."

Thanks for checking in and a happy V.D. [Valentine's Day] to you too!

xo

eg

I e-mail back to Ellyn:

Date: Monday, 20 Feb, 2006
To: eg336
From richardson
Subject: re: I'm in Australia

Ellyn—thanks for your e-mail—i'm keen on staying in touch. . . .
But I am glad to be "half a world away" from the turmoils at home. . . .
The geographic cure.

g'day, I

I'm not quite through my e-mail when I hear Maisie tapping on my door.

It is twelve o'clock. I wave her in. We hug. She's a cheerful presence.

"Are your ready to go for a little coffee?" she asks. "We can firm up your schedule."

I grab my take-away lunch, and we walk to one of the outdoor coffee shops that are sprinkled about the campus, this one a seven-minute "short" walk from my office. The temperature is rising.

For my fellowship I had agreed to do two workshops, meet with a few Ph.D. students, and give a communitywide lecture. But so many requests have come in for my time and so many venues sound interesting that I succumb to the overscheduling of my Oz life. I insist, though, on one week totally free so I can do some traveling.

I return to my office and e-mail a note with my Oz schedule to Betty's daughter.

Date: Mon, Feb 20, 2006
To: pksmith
From: richardson
Subject: Please give to Betty

Penny—please print and give to Betty. Hope all's well with you/yours and her. Thanks.

Betty—I hope you're feeling better. . . . I love being in my own office with a great computer and tech support. I've missed that. Ernest is set up in his studio . . . he's a happy camper.

Here's my schedule for Melbourne. There will be the unscheduled, of course, too. Dear me—what have I gotten myself into? Why do I have to work so damn much? Yes, I know, I've brought it upon myself. No one else to blame but ME. Just being with people is so much work for me, I'm such an introvert. God, what if I had to shop, cook, and clean up too? Good that I'm living in "assisted living."

Love, I

LAUREL'S MELBOURNE SCHEDULE

Tues, 2/21: Meet with Lynda S. (Arts Centre) to plan work with artists; meet with Ph.D. students

Wed, 2/22: Meet with Anne W. to visit the Sisters of Mercy project on indigenous narratives

Thurs, 2/23: Critical discourse group workshop

Fri, 2/24: Meet with group of Ph.D. students; meet with individual Ph.D.students; dinner with ethnographic drama group at University House

Sat, 2/25: Dinner at Maisie's (Trevor coming too)

Mon, 2/26: Artistic and creative faculty colloquia and workshop

Tues, 2/27: Arts Centre (9-6),"Telling Lives" workshop

Wed, 2/28: Artistic and creative faculty dinner, University Club

Thurs-Mon, 3/1-3/6: LAUREL FREE TO TRAVEL OZ

Tues, 3/7: Lunch and conference with Julianne re rewriting of three textbooks; conferences with Ph.D. students

Wed 3/8: Lecture and meeting with Laura B. at RMIT; meetings with urban Aboriginal Ph.D. students

Thurs, 3/9: Distinguished lecture and dinner

Fri, 3/10: SHOPPING WITH MAISIE!!!

Mon, 3/13: Meet with Maisie re her union case; High Table at University College

Tues 3/14: Meet with Maisie and Trevor re writing of proposal for textbook, conferences in America, publishing venues; high tea with Ernest, Trevor, and Maisie; High Table at University College

Wed: 3/15: Fly to Sydney

It is 3 p.m., and a smiling Maisie is knocking on my door. It's time for me to meet Dean Kingsley, his secretaries and assistants, and Maisie's colleagues: Peter, Paul, and Mary. No: Peter, Paul, and Trevor. Trevor's genial, warm, and witty. I think he and Ernest will be chums. At 4:30 I retrace my route back to my apartment. Forty minutes later I arrive and take a power nap. I wake up coughing and wheezing. My head hurts. It is too late to call Betty.

Ernest limps in, enthused about his painting of Port Arthur's penal colony. He's chosen an angle that foregrounds a ruined arch in the prison walls through which the viewer can see a small bridge leading to a green pasture. We walk to our first dinner at University College and seat ourselves with visitors from Singapore, England, Canada, Japan, and France. Several resident advisors—graduate students from the United Kingdom—join us. The Delhian chef, trained in Paris, has prepared three different dinners: meat, vegetarian, vegan. I engage in politely awkward small talk with the others at my table.

At the other tables members of the student welcoming committee are teaching the new students the college song, whose refrain is an enthusiastic "F**k 'em!" No one at our table seems to notice but Ernest and me.

We skip coffee and tea in the Common Room and head back to our apartment. We want to watch a little telly before we call it a night. Which of the three channels shall it be? 1990s *Law and Order*? *Dancing with the (Aussie) Stars*? Cricket?

Tuesday, February 21

"I'll have to take back my apnea machine," I tell Ernest in the morning. I have barely slept and my lungs feel as if they're going to expand out of my body.

"Of course," he says. "It's your machine."

I feel guilty taking back "my machine" because his sleep apnea is severe, and mine is borderline, induced by allergies. But if I don't get some sleep, I'll be an ogre.

"You can use it tomorrow night," I say. "We'll take turns."

I try to call Betty but no one answers. I hope Mike has taken her to the casino.

"Good morning," I say to Dean Kingsley, as I pass his open door. My anxiety around administrators surfaces as I wonder if he is wondering why I am coming to "work" so late. With the grace and speed of a greyhound, Kingsley, dressed in a gray silk suit, bounds out of his office into the hall to greet me. Because of the heat I am wearing a short, lime green cotton knit dress with magenta and blue fish flying all over it. Being underdressed adds to my nervousness.

"What a lovely shirt and tie," I say, taking the attention off me and off any ideas he might have that I am a fashion schlump. In America my comment might be construed as sexual harassment.

"Thank you," Kingsley says. "I chose the fabrics in Thailand and had them fashioned to my specifications."

"Very nice," I say.

"Here's the brochure for your lecture," Kingsley says, looking very pleased.

The brochure features Kingsley, complete with his photograph and bio. Two scant lines provide the title, time, and place of my lecture. My name is there too.

I walk to my office and do my e-mail. There's Ellyn again, bless her.

From: eg336
To: richardson
Subject: Re: re/you/betty

Betty was thrilled (!) to get your call. She said that you sounded better than you had in years. Mike was over watching the Olympics with her. Good on ya for calling!

xo

Mary picks me up at the office and we walk thirty minutes to the Sisters of Mercy. The day unfolds. I am back in the apartment at four. I reach Betty. She had been to the doctor earlier in the day. She is coughing. She has her third new aide, and second visiting nurse.

"This is how old I am," Betty says. "I asked the nurse about urine leakage when I cough and she told me to use sanitary pads. I looked at her like she was nuts. I was envisioning an elastic strap around my waist and metal hooks!"

Betty had a hysterectomy almost forty years ago. After nine miscarriages, she told her husband, Joe, "That's enough. We'll adopt." They registered with a Jewish adoption agency, and soon along came Penny.

"A bluebird just flew by my window," Betty says. She's coughing. "My daddy's watching over me."

She saw a bluebird on a tree in her backyard the day her father died.

Thursday, February 23

My writing workshop with the critical discourse group was scheduled for today. I was exhausted going in. My inner compass is out of whack as I am not yet adjusted to the Southern Hemisphere's magnetism, shadows, movement of the sun. My nighttime body gasps and moans, and my daytime one aches from the walking. My mind overflows with people, ideas, challenges, and my introverted self feels abandoned. I can't breathe at night and I worry about Betty's incessant coughing.

"My twin desire is that my writing be both artful and true," I said to the assembled group.

"Is that why you experiment with different formats and styles?" someone asked.

"That's right. By using different formats—prose, poetry, dialogue, drama—you learn different things about your subject."

"What are you working on now, Laurel?" a different someone asked.

What *was* I working on? Two years ago Ernest's and my coauthored book, *Travels with Ernest,* had been published. Since then I seem to have been working on *not* working, but that was not the answer I could give to this workshop. How embarrassing would that be!

What was I working on? My eyes went into their "I'm thinking" mode—first a squint, then widened and looking to the uppermost left above and beyond the people and objects in the room as though an answer was there in the furthermost corner of the room—or in my unconscious.

Aha! I *was* diligently working on my Daybook. I was writing a *book*. And because my creative process is not complete until the creation has an audience, I knew at that moment that just writing the Daybook, perhaps reading it to my memoir writing group, would not complete my process. I would want my Daybook published.

"I'm using the daybook format—dialogue, scenes, e-mails, memoir—to write a book about the dying of my best friend," I said. I felt an inexplicable relief.

"Does your friend know you are writing this book?" another someone asked.

"No," I said, without adding that I didn't know I was either until this past moment. I thought about the slipperiness of friendship, writing, research, and situational ethics.

"Are you going to tell her?" a different another someone asked.

"I don't know what's the right thing to do," I answered. "Not telling her about the Daybook gives me the freedom to write without harming her or censuring myself. Telling her might affect what she says to me. Much worse, it might hurt her. I'm not sure if I'm acting rightly or not."

Following the workshop I decide to send an upbeat e-mail to Betty, my family, and friends.

Subject: greetings to friends and family

Dear EVERYONE,

Life is good.

Maybe that is all I need to say. . . . Well of course there is more. Fresh fruit and veggies, warm-hearted people with the graciousness of our southern women, and the laid-backness and friendliness of our midwestern ones.

I am working hard here though—so many different kinds of workshops and people wanting to talk with me—I had no idea I had influenced so wide a range of persons, and I am humbled and flattered and surprised.

I am being treated like a rock star!

It is wonderful to write this little bit to you all, knowing I won't be expected to do anything other than be who I am.

On the weekend Ernest and I will go to Healesville, a sanctuary for wild animals, . . . and we'll go to several art galleries in the Yarra Valley. . . . Dinner at Maisie's house! On Sunday we'll explore the "famous" Lygnon Street shops and restaurants.

Cheers and love from way down under, Mom/Grandma/Laurel

I push the send button.

Friday, February 24
TGIF!!!

Saturday, February 25
Dinner at Maisie's was the most sumptuous dinner I ever had in someone's home. Because the night was so hot, Maisie prepared a cold dinner for eight. She set out plates of chilled shrimp, crab legs, and oysters, and bowls of green salads, a variety of green and black olives, and French and rye breads with three kinds of butter. I thought this was our dinner, and I filled up. But that was only what Ozzies call the "entre." Maisie cleared the table and put out the "main," two platters of cold sliced tenderloin, one rare and one medium, three sauces, bowls of vinegared potato salad and creamy potato salad, plates of baby asparagus, green, red, and yellow marinated peppers, garden-ripened heritage tomatoes sprinkled with parmesan cheese, and popover biscuits. Then she served three desserts—a lemon meringue tartlet, chocolate mousse, and Mum's summer pudding. I declined the after-dessert dessert—sorbets and creams, coffees and teas, cashews and minties.

On the way back from Maisie's, I think about Betty's relationship to food. She likes upscale restaurants, interesting spices, and meat. There was a time when I would have called her a good eater.

Thirty years ago a mutual friend asked me if Betty were bulimic. I'd never seen any concrete evidence of an eating disorder, only that she was very thin, smoked, and had a mortal fear of being fat. In her mid-fifties, stomach acids had destroyed her teeth, a common pattern in bulimia. "Don't pull them all out," I had cautioned her. But she thought it was the best thing to do. If Betty was bulimic, she held this card very close.

Betty is secretive and discreet too. She keeps her words under control, never letting her secrets or confidences slip out, rarely gossiping. She can absolutely be trusted to keep private matters private. She feels she can absolutely trust me too. Do I have a right to reveal her life? Cast possible aspersions upon it? Or, contrarily, would she be relieved to know that her struggles with food and illnesses would at last be made public, so others might know how brave a woman she really had been or even be helped in their own struggles by her story?

This much I do know about myself, though. If Betty had told me in confidence that she had an eating disorder, I would not be writing about it. Just as I do not write about some other things.

Sunday, February 26

"Hi, Jessica." I am talking to my sister on the phone. It's early Sunday afternoon in Melbourne and early Saturday evening in Des Moines, where she lives. Ernest and I have returned early from our Lygnon Street expedition because of the impossible heat (108 degrees Fahrenheit), directional mixups, and threatening weather.

"We're having a monsoon here!" I tell her. "Where our windows meet, water is pouring in."

"You better get some towels," she says. My sister loves to solve problems.

"Ernest," I yell. He's in the living room. "Can you bring some towels? We have a leak."

"Yikes," I say to my sister. "Now the ceiling is leaking. Water is pouring onto the desk."

Ernest comes in with towels. He surveys the rising water level on the floor and announces, "It's Niagara Falls!"

"Did you hear that?" I say to Jessica.

"Yes."

I like that she's part of my adventure.

"Honey," Ernest says, "I think we can use that phone to better advantage right now."

"Okay," I say. "Talk to you later, Jessica. Love ya."

Ernest empties drawers, clears shelves and closet, and carries everything of ours into the center of the living room, hoping the roof there will not succumb to the deluge. I call every number I find in my *Guide to University College* brochure. There is no one on duty at Reception. There is no emergency phone number. There is over two inches of water on the soaked carpet. I phone the last number on the list and "just happen" to find a resident advisor in the Common Room where the phone is ringing.

"Would you like me to bring some more towels?" she asks.

"It's way past towels," I say. "You need a sucking machine."

I can hardly breathe.

"The water is filthy too," I say, looking at the brown stains on my feet. "You need more than a sucking machine. You need a new rug. Maybe a new floor."

Then I realize that this is not the first time this rug has been inundated with rain. Indeed, the lingering noxious smell and toxic air can be traced to the mildew and mold growing wild for years in this apartment.

By late Sunday afternoon we are ensconced in a different apartment about the size of one of those hotel suite bargains you get on the Internet and are sorry about later. It's on the first floor and its carpet is wet too, but less so than in other available apartments. A cleaning crew arrives with sucking machines, but no one is talking about replacing rugs. No one is talking about fixing the downspouts either. The only phone is tethered to a wall plate in the hallway. The cord is too short to reach the couch. I bring a dining chair over and set the phone on it, turn kitty-corner on the couch seat, scrunching my hip, and try to call Betty. She doesn't answer.

Ernest uses my CPAP in the smelly, mildewed bedroom. I sleep on blankets on the hallway's linoleum floor.

Monday, February 27

To: richardson
From: eg336
Subject: Betty

Betty went into the hospital Friday night. Penny says that she is still way better than last October. It continues to be 2 steps forward, 1 step back. Hopefully, she'll be home in the next couple of days.

xo

To: eg336
From: richardson
Subject: Betty

Ellyn—thanks for your e-mail. Do you know which hospital? Do you have her phone number?

Cheers, I

Tuesday, February 28

I am sitting at my desk in my office in Alice Hoy Hall. Ellyn has e-mailed me that she doesn't know the name of the hospital. Soon I will be facilitating a workshop for the artistic and creative education faculty. My exhaustion is palpable.

Think, Laurel, think. Remember the name of the hospital. I close my eyes, nod off. *Kent! It's Kent Hospital in Dover, Delaware.* I remember how weird it seemed when Betty was sick in Dover once before—maybe twice—she ended up in Kent. *You might even have that hospital's phone number in your travel address book,* I say sotto voce, conspiratorially. When I am really tired, I talk to myself as if I am another person, a person who needs to be cajoled, encouraged, calmed down, and convinced to take action. I do have the number and I call Betty. She has pneumonia and explosive diarrhea. She'll be in the hospital for a spell.

"I'm going on a holiday next week," I tell her. "We're going to drive the Great Ocean Road to Port Fairy. I may not be able to reach you by phone."

"I know," Betty says. "I'm so glad you're getting to do this. Keep notes. Write a lot."

"I'll have lots of stories," I say.

"Stories, . . ." Betty sounds pensive. "I've lost so much. I can't remember anything. And now I'm even forgetting my stories."

"Write them," I say.

"You're the writer," she counters. "You write them."

"Would you like me to?" I ask.

"Yes. Tell the world about me."

I facilitate the five-hour workshop and walk back to the apartment, totally worn out. My nerves are frayed, my body is shaking. I don't think I ever want to work again. I yell at Ernest about something. I think I am going to have a nervous breakdown.

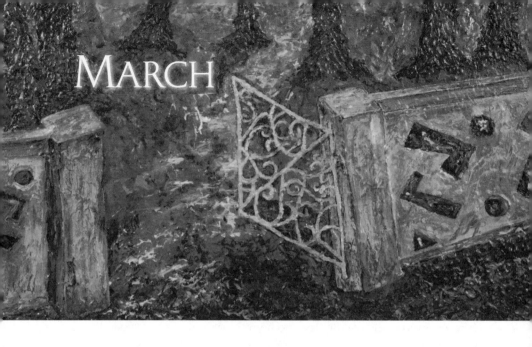

MARCH

Friday to Sunday, March 3 to 5

Port Fairy is magical. Here at the confluence of the South Pacific and Indian oceans I can breathe. Everywhere I want to go is an easy walk from our historic hotel, a Comfort Inn (!), newly refurbished with faux marble and stainless steel. No mold or mildew. Ernest props his ailing foot on a garden stool outside our room while I strike off on my own, relishing my independence.

When I walk about with problems on my mind, I look for "signs" that might help me work through those problems. On my mind now is how to let go of my identity as a professor of sociology so I can move on in my life. I happen upon the Port Fairy Bookstore, a boxcar-size store owned by a taciturn man who chooses not to speak to me. I return the favor. Maybe what he has shelved under sociology will be a sign. I commit the titles to memory:

> *Time Illusion*
> *Having It All*
> *Living and Loving Together: Contracts That Work*
> *A Child's Guide to the Crime Factory*
> *The Joy of Twins*

Sounds and Society
How to Discipline with Love
Decorating with Finesse
Guide to Midyears Career
New Testament
A Path to Perfection
The Private Future

If there is a sign here, it's that I should expand my idea of what constitutes a life in sociology. I'd like to talk about that with Betty, but I don't think she'd be up to it anymore. I file the thought away.

Later Ernest and I, wrapped in each other's warmth, sit on a rock on Griffith Island and watch the sun set. When have we ever done this before—sat quietly together for two hours? Just as darkness descends, we see and hear what we have come for. Thousands of shearwater bird pairs swoop back from the ocean with fish for their little ones waiting, hungry, in their burrows. Whoosh—whoosh—whoosh—and then silence, and then all over the island, "Cheepity-cheep-cheep cheep."

Each November the shearwaters fly fifteen thousand miles from the Aleutian Islands to Griffith Island. Mated for life, pairs fix their burrow for their single egg. Once it is laid, the pair flies off for a bit, returning when the egg hatches. For the next six months the parents fly away at daybreak and return at nightfall with bounty for their chick. In late March all the parents fly fifteen thousand miles back to the Aleutians, leaving the babies behind. About two weeks later, hungry fledglings emerge from their burrows. "Where's Mom? Where's Dad?" they must be wondering. "Ah, they've flown back to the Aleutians. We'd better join them." And so the fledglings fly by themselves the fifteen thousand miles "back" to a place they've never been.

Are the shearwaters a sign too? A sign that I can fly away and survive? A sign that I can go "back" to where I have never been?

Monday, March 6

We're back in our apartment in Melbourne. It's about a week since I've talked to Betty. When she doesn't answer her home phone, I call Delaware's Kent Hospital. That's where she was when I last called.

"I'd like to talk to Betty Kirschner," I tell the operator. "She's a patient, I think."

"No one by that name here," the operator says.

"Are you sure?"

"How do you spell it?"

"It's Kirschner," I say, "K-i-r-s-c-h-n-e-r."

"Krishna?"

"No, *Kirschner*."

"Oh, Christner."

"No, K-i-r-s-c-h-n-e-r."

"Oh, Kirschner. . . . How do you spell the first name?"

"B-e-t-t-y."

"Oh. *Missus* Kirschner."

"I guess."

"I'll connect you," says the operator.

"Hi, Betty," I say. "How's it goin'?"

"Not doing so well. Twelve days I've been here. I have diarrhea."

"Probably from the heavy-duty antibiotics for the pneumonia," I offer. "Have you thought of taking probiotics? They're natural."

I've had this conversation with Betty innumerable times over the years. She's refused probiotics, homeopathics, or any OTCs that might settle her digestive track, relieve pains in her joints, or reduce her anxiety. I recall how disappointed she always is when slews of medical tests in and out of the hospital find "nothing wrong."

Now Betty announces, "They want to do some tests for cancer. But I have to leave the hospital and come back to get them."

"That's weird," I say.

"Everything's weird. It's a hospital," Betty continues. "They've only given me an MRI and esophageal test. I don't know the results. Does it matter? They want me to order a GI consult."

"Are you going to do *that*?"

"It'll give me something to do."

"How's Penny?" I ask.

"Penny hasn't brought me daffodils. They're available in the store and she hasn't brought them."

"Have you asked her to bring some?"

"No!"

"Asking isn't the same," I agree.

"If I were home in Kent everybody would be bringing me daffodils. The house would be full of them. Flowers are not part of caretaking here, not part of giving when someone's in the hospital. Back in October the pulmonologist told me I'd never see another daffodil. I guess my daughter is making that prediction come true!"

"The doctor meant, if you didn't stop smoking."

"No, smoking didn't matter. Penny doesn't hear things that have to get done," Betty says.

"I'm sorry."

"Penny did bring bulbs."

"Bulbs?"

"Yes, daffodil bulbs. In a little pot."

"That was nice," I say. "Different. Something for the future."

Someone enters Betty's room.

"Not that!" she yells. "I told you I wanted decaf tea. Hot!"

And then to me, a bit proudly, "I've pissed off that nurse."

I wonder if "*Missus Kirschner*" also pissed off the operator.

Tuesday, March 7

I awake after a fitful night, labored breathing, and nightmares. In one nightmare, after I have worked hard preparing a writing workshop, I discover that the students are hundreds of the elderly. They reject my plans. They want something more personal, intimate, and psychological. From the dais I improvise, "Ah . . . think about something in your life that mattered to you—something that has moved you." The students begin leaving, chattering among themselves as they go. Nothing has mattered. They have been moved by nothing.

Wednesday, March 8

"I'm not getting paid for my work here," I say to Betty. She's still in the hospital.

"What?"

"When I arrived there was six thousand dollars Australian in my account, but when I asked Maisie about it yesterday she said it was all gone."

"Where did it go?"

"Well, Dean Kingsley has taken five thousand dollars for the dinner after my lecture. And maybe he's charging for my office space and computer help."

"Tsk-tsk. When money gets into a dean's pocket, it never gets out."

"Isn't it the damndest thing?"

"Well, at least you can look forward to a spectacular dinner."

Thursday, March 9
University College, UniMelb, Melbourne AU

Dear Betty,

Well, my primary reason for being in Melbourne—to give the Distinguished Lecture—is now over! Surprisingly, I'm not too tired. Actually, I'm a-buzz.

The Internet service (i.e., e-mail) is down and it's too late to phone you. But I wanted to share my experience—so being the resourceful Laurel that you have come to know and love, I have commandeered a computer in the Common Room that (Yeah!) has Word on it. I even have access to an HP printer. And paper at five cents per sheet ("very reasonable for Oz," the resident advisor tells me). So here comes a snail mail to you. I'll have the pleasure of sharing with you now something you might read next month.

Five hundred people filled the stadium-style auditorium, the largest turnout ever for the lecture series. I was in a pit (but not the pits) at the front of the room, without drinking water, but wired for sound and camera. My benefactors, Lord Esky and Lady Katherine Turnbull, sat in the second row. Lord Esky looks like the old Esquire man—bulging eyes, shiny white skin, hair, and goatee. Lady Katherine, largish and pretty, looks like a member of the horsey set that went to Penny's fancy girl's school.

"Writing for Your Life" was my topic. I talked about my car accident and coma, and how writing helped my recovery. I read some, spoke some, walked about. As you know, I am a theater person at heart—like you, a bit show-offy and always exhilarated by moving an audience to action, tears, or laughter. Everyone laughed at the concluding story of my recent CAT scan and the radiologist's astonishment that I was as old as I am because I had a "perfect brain."

At the close of the lecture, a dapper Dean Kingsley, with great flourish and gusto, handed me a little black velvet bag. Inside was a little black "University of Melbourne" clock (made in China). "So you can always remember us," he said. Surreptitiously I looked for a check—in vain. "I give this clock to all our visitors," Kingsley tells the audience. "Isn't it elegant?" I feel some sympathy for Dean Kingsley. This is his first deanship, his first-ever university position. Handing me the gift, he looks like a pleased little boy, waiting for a pat on the head.

Ten of us—Lord and Lady Turnbull, Maisie, Dean Kingsley, Anne (a royal on her mother's side), Jack, the official representative of UniMelb's chancellor (who was himself meeting with the Parliament as I spoke), two other administrators, Ernest, and I retired to the Queen's Room at "the Club." I was glad Maisie was there. She's becoming a friend. Actually, she's a sweetheart.

Dean Kingsley seated me between Lord Esky and himself, he seated Lady Katherine across from me flanking Ernest on the left, Anne-the-royal he seated flanking his right, and at the table's hinter regions he seated the Designated Lesser Souls.

"What wine would you like?" Kingsley asks me, perusing the extensive wine list.

"Ernest and I don't drink," I say. "It makes us too tired the next day."

"That's un-Australian," objects Lord Esky.

Kingsley orders eight bottles of wine at $100.00 a whack.

"Call me 'Esky,'" Lord Esky says.

"Call me 'Laurel,'" I say.

Esky chuckles. "Tell me, then, Laurel, what are two things that have most negatively surprised you about Australia?"

I like Esky and besides, I don't want to bite the hand that's feeding me, so I demur for a bit, but Esky persists, commanding me to answer.

"There are no bathtubs," I say.

"Come to our house," Lady Katherine says. "Esky thought I was overdoing it, but I have a large bathtub in our house. I spend hours in it. Reading. What else is there to do?"

"Humph," says Esky.

Esky pours wine into my empty wineglass. "I won't allow you to remain un-Australian," he says, topping off his wineglass.

"Show everyone the clock I gave you," Kingsley commands me.

The clock reaches Ernest, who examines it earnestly. "It's not working," he says.

"What? How can that be?" Kingsley is bereft. "I've given the same clock to everyone who visits. I've never had a problem. I'll get it repaired."

Kingsley has a knack for making me feel special.

Kingsley's turns his attention to capturing Lord Esky's. Kingsley has a plan to market his college and wants Esky to serve on a "consultation board." Kingsley talks through me. I might as well be invisible. I sit back in my chair and smile at Ernest.

"Prince Phillip is arriving tomorrow," Lady Katherine says in a loud voice. "For the dreadful Commonwealth Games. Esky is having lunch with him. I am not going. It is so boring."

"You weren't invited," Esky booms back.

Esky turns his attention to me. "There must be something besides the lack of bathtubs that you find less than good about Australia," he says.

I take a long breath and go for it. "One thing I find really troublesome is the lack of facilities for people with disabilities."

Esky pulls back. He did not expect this answer. I am not going to restrain myself. He asked for it, so he'll get it.

"In all the time I have been in Australia," I begin slowly, conversationally, "I have seen only one fellow on crutches and two people in wheelchairs."

Then my internal rhetorician takes over. "If you are in a wheelchair, on crutches, or simply challenged by a sore foot or aging limbs, forget leaving your house. Forget about getting a university education. Or a job. Or a meal! Or a coffee, for goodness sake! Sidewalks, trams, street crossings, building doors—none of them disability-friendly. And then there are the restrooms, inaccessible down flights of steps in dark corridors, sometimes several blocks away from where you are dining." I take a breath and conclude. "There is almost nothing that makes your country available to those who are permanently or temporarily physically limited. That's a big negative."

You'd have been proud of me, Betty. I was thinking of you—and how you could not have gotten around in Australia at all, and I was thinking of Ernest, and how difficult this has been for him with his injured foot, and I was thinking of myself and how physically challenged that I—a healthy and able but aging woman—have been. Until forced by Esky, I hadn't realized how scandalously backward I thought Australia was regarding their infirm and aged. Australia could never be <u>my place.</u>

"We're doing some things," Kingsley jumps in, obviously embarrassed by my rant. "It's too expensive, though."

"Well, let's talk about smoking," Esky says. "I'm against smoking."

"Ernest and I quit twenty-five years ago," I say.

"How did you accomplish that?"

"We had tried quitting separately, but that had never worked. I knew that if I started smoking again, Ernest would too. I quit smoking because I loved Ernest."

"That's absurd," says Esky. No namby-pamby lord here. "Only a wife would talk that way. I bet Ernest wouldn't give that reason." Ernest is deeply immersed in conversation with Katherine when Esky calls across the table, "Ernest, I have a quiz for you. Why did you quit smoking? (a) I was smoking at the petrol station, (b) I couldn't find my way through the smoke-filled corridors of my country's political back rooms, (c) my lit cigarette torched a heritage farmhouse."

"Well, actually—," Ernest begins our familiar conarrated story of how we came to be ex-smokers, but Esky interrupts him.

LAST WRITES

"Just get to the chase," he says.

"You'd better get it right," Jack-the-rep. interjects. "Your marriage depends on it."

"I quit because I love Laurel," Ernest says.

"I cannot believe you actually said that," Esky stammers. He is visibly taken aback.

"I don't love Esky," Katherine volunteers. "It bothers him, but it's true."

"Ernest can be totally outrageous," I say. "But I stay with him. That must prove I love him."

"That's just the entertainment factor," she says. "You can love a book or a cat. You can't love a spouse."

Everyone focuses on Katherine.

"Esky is a serial flatterer," she continues. "He has a crush now on Vicky, the principal at Trent College. But poor Esky. Vicky has a crush on my father."

"I think you know Vicky," a smiling Esky says to Kingsley.

"I do," Kingsley agrees. "Charming woman. She helped my daughter achieve a first in cycling." Kingsley then slides into his athletic achievements in the upper-crust sport of rowing, his daughter's in rowing and cycling, his son's in—well, in everything, I think.

"So Anne," Esky says, "How is your mother?"

"She's doing fine," Anne-daughter-of-royal says.

"Remember me to her," Esky says. He is gleaming. "Remember me to her," he repeats. "Tell her I remember fondly our time alone in the swimming pool. She'll remember."

The "serial flatterer" then turns to me. But instead of flattering me, Esky begins a diatribe on what's wrong with America. "And Bush went to war without the consent of the U.N. So he is just like Hitler."

Across the table Lady Katherine and Ernest engage in a similar conversation. Later Ernest tells me Lady Katherine declared that "Israel should be wiped off the map."

Lady Katherine tells us that Prince Charles gave Di seven books to take on their honeymoon and instructed her to read one each day so they'd have something to talk about at dinner, and that this was not idle gossip because Katherine's old schoolmate's ex-nanny was told about it by Prince Charles's nanny, and Ernest says, "The crown had to sacrifice a virgin," and Lord Esky says, "Humph!," and Anne and Maisie burst out laughing, and Jack-the-rep. menacingly slashes the air with his dessert knife, and then Ernest says, "Everyone in Australia comes from a line of convicts," and Kingsley shouts, "What's wrong with that?"

So "My Dinner with Lord Esky" drew to a speedy close.

Kingsley surreptitiously pens his name on the half-full bottles of wine, on the lowboy behind his chair. I overhear him whisper to our waiter, "I'll get them tomorrow. Recork them. No reason for them to go to waste."

Oh, Betty, you would have had a blast. Social-class networks superimposed on the academic ones. You'd have been a great dinner partner, but I'm afraid Kingsley would have seated you in the hallway.

Tomorrow I'm off on a shopping spree with Maisie.

I hope when this letter reaches you that you're feeling good. Thanks for being the person I write for—my favorite first listener.

Love,
Laurel

P.S. As we were leaving, Anne (whose mother Lord Esky had drawn through the mud, well, the pool), says there was a scandal about Lord Esky that she'd tell us about later. I hope it's a juicy one.

My letter to Betty finished, I go back to the apartment. Ernest is still awake, and we rehash our "Dinner with Esky."

Ernest says, "If you hadn't quit smoking twenty-five years ago, you wouldn't be here in Australia now, writing to Betty. You'd both be dying."

Friday, March 10

Maisie and I are in Fitzroy's on Brunswick Street, where Maisie is buying jeans and a snazzy red and black striped T-shirt with a square neck cut low to her bosom. She looks smashing. Blaring into my ears is ungodly American music: *G**damn your eyes, go to hell, g**damn your eyes.*

No one else seems to notice. We stop at the homoeopathic store where *Jesus Christ Superstar* blasts. A Max Factor Certified Cosmetologist, wearing an apron emblazoned with a transfer print of Michelangelo's David complete with genitalia, offers her services. I decline. This might be 1970s America.

"May I try on these earrings?" I ask the earring designer at the Little Salon.

"It's not allowed," she says. Elvis is singing "Heartbreak Hotel."

"In America," I begin, and then stop myself. "I'll take them."

She places the earrings in a round plastic case with "love/hate" printed on the liner paper. I remember the times when Betty and I went earring shopping in Sedona. We had three criteria for choosing earrings—weight, length, and authenticity. Once Betty convinced me to spend the $100 the Navajo trader wanted for a longish tin, bone, and turquoise pair. She said she'd buy them from me if I decided later that I didn't like them. She's not been able to wear earrings for years, though. Something about allergies or vasculitis or something. There's always something. The earrings I am buying here—red jewelry wire pierced through red Australian glass, not too heavy and not too long, handmade by the woman wrapping them up—meet all three of our earring criteria.

Maisie seems agitated when she tells me, "My supervisor thinks it is so gross that you are not getting paid for all the work you've done here that he's going to find somewhere at least a thousand dollars."

"That's very nice," I say.

"I hope this money issue hasn't affected our relationship," she says.

"Of course not." I give Maisie a big hug.

I'm easy about money issues and so are most of the people in my life—my family, Betty, the memoir writing group, and now Maisie. My ex-dean was not. When we would go to lunch, she'd figure out her portion of the bill to the penny and then tip the waitperson a precise 15 percent, before taxes. It's embarrassing to see pennies on the table. One can learn a lot about another over a little bill.

"Do you want to go shopping again tomorrow?" Maisie asks.

"Indeed I do."

"We'll go to the Rose Street Art Market. And we'll invite Ernest."

"He probably won't want to come—he gets bored at art markets."

"But he can come and drink some coffee."

I am so happy I have a woman friend here in Melbourne.

Saturday, March 11

"There, I found you," I say to Betty. As usual, when I can't reach her at home, I try the hospital. "How come you're back there?"

"It got boring. I got pneumonia. It doesn't seem to be clearing up. It doesn't show on the x-ray. Doctor One said, 'There's nothing wrong with you. Go home!' Doctor Two said, 'Stay.'"

"Good thing you're not a dog."

"Penny's supposed to be going to a major seminar this week but she's not going."

"So you can follow Doctor One's orders and go home, Lassie."

"No. Penny will be at work some of the time, and Mike doesn't want to be with me when she's not there. He doesn't want to be with me when I change clothes. That doesn't please me."

Her breath is halting. I think I hear her thinking.

"I keep remembering a conversation we've had off and on, about the importance of writing," Betty says. "Mortality rests in getting your name in print."

"I think you mean *immortality*," I say.

"Yes. Immortality only comes from having your name in print. You've always denied that, Laurel. Now there you are going around the world. Write me an obit. Write my story, the forgotten stories. My life is my *story*, and now almost none of my stories are written down. I can't remember them now. Just more letting go."

"I'll write your stories," I say. "And the story of our friendship."

"That would please me," Betty says.

"Even if I write about the rough spots?"

"I'll chance it."

Sunday, March 12

I am so tired of working and yet I can't let it go. I want to say: *This is it! I'm done! Let my previous work do the working.* All the cheers, flowers, and accolades don't make up for my desire to be done with it all. Why can't I let it go?

People want me to help them. I can't help anyone. I am so tired.

Here comes the death of a friend.

I can let go.

Monday, March 13

My last day at the office. My little black clock is on my desk in its little black bag. I write my thank-you notes and do a final check of my e-mail. Anne-the-royal has sent me news items about Lord Esky. After fifteen years of litigation the Supreme Court acquitted him of investment fraud charges but said its decision didn't necessarily mean he was innocent. To the press Lord Esky announced, "I've never doubted my innocence."

No wonder Dean Kingsley summarily ended our dinner when Ernest mentioned Aussies-as-convicts.

I print out my e-mails, clear my computer, gather up my office stuff, and begin my last trek across campus to my apartment. The walk has become easier.

"Look at this," I say, showing Ernest Anne's e-mail.

"Well," he says, "nobody's perfect."

Tuesday, March 14

"I have a thought," Ernest says to me in the morning before we are to leave Melbourne. He's responding to my dispiritedness.

"Being here for you has been like being back in the sociology department at Ohio State University. A department you left because you couldn't deal with it anymore."

He has my full attention.

"Allergies—that's Ohio State."

Due to a faulty architectural design, my office had been the sole recipient of the ozone from Cop-EZ, the sole copying center for the university's six thousand professors, and sixty-five thousand students. The two persons who had occupied the office before me had died of cancer. I couldn't breathe in that office.

"Physical challenges—that's Ohio State."

My teaching and classroom assignments required me to walk half miles or more in rain, snow, sleet, and hail carrying pounds of paper—syllabi, handouts, student papers, lecture notes, books.

"Great teaching begetting too much teaching—that's Ohio State."

One year I taught about a thousand undergraduates and fifty graduate students, and served on three honors thesis and twelve dissertation committees.

"Screwed by administrators—that's Ohio State."

My dean denigrating my research and writing.

"Underpaid—that's Ohio State."

I left the department as a full professor in rank for sixteen years making but a scant more than the assistant professor they hired to replace me.

After this conversation, I feel invigorated.

Wednesday, March 15

Time to pack, clean up, think. I bring the bright red flowers in the bright green box, a gift from the critical discourse group, to the Common Room. Maisie tells me that the check for my honorarium has been drawn, but that Kingsley refuses to sign it. He wants to find out about "protocol." I do have my clock. It's fixed.

"How're you doing today?" I ask Betty. She's home from the hospital.

"Doing better," she says. "You learn things when you're away from home. I've rediscovered that I like living alone."

"Why's that?"

"Things get their places and stay there! I feel dissed here. People don't do things the way I do!"

"Do you have your daffodils yet?"

"Ha! A couple bulbs are sprouting but there are no flowers! This is a lifestyle we know nothing about. Penny's friends and family work all the time and then roam from house to house doing nothing . . . stand around, drink beer, clear out the woods. Very, very odd. Very male. Rural. Very throwback. Not total throwback—everyone has to have a new pickup. . . . Everyone knows everyone from kindergarten. . . . No content in their talk, but a lot of doing for each other."

Their lives sound not so bad to me.

"Betty, we're in Sydney," I say on the phone. "Been here two days!"

"Is it beautiful?" she asks.

"Our Elizabeth Avenue apartment is nice, in a 1920s kind of way. Lovely view of a boat dock, roof gardens, and a cricket field. Then there's our neighborhood."

"Yes?"

"A police station on our corner, and down the street drug dealers, boy and girl prostitutes, gay clubs, massage parlors, triple-X theaters."

"Have you been to the Opera House?"

"Yeah, and back again."

Having been shown the way and told it was a short walk, Ernest and I guilelessly went on our way through the red-light district, down two hundred granite steps to a thruway that we jaywalked to reach a freight boat harbor that tailed into a hilly city park that led, after a mile, into the Sydney Bay Walkway, which in a half mile reached the hundred granite steps that led into the Opera House. The walk took nearly ninety minutes. It was blistering hot. Ernest stumbled around, keeping a stiff upper lip. Inside the Opera House, I recoiled. It felt like the bowels of Ohio State University's football stadium. We declined the partial-view opera tickets, each costing three hundred dollars Australian. Only a few thousand more feet, and down some fifty stairs, and at last we reached our *new* destination—the loo.

Finding no cabs, trains, or buses that would return us to Elizabeth Street, and being advised of such at the Visitor Center, we walked back the way we had come, both of us stumbling this time.

"I think Aussies always say something is a 'short walk' because 'you can't get there from here' on public transportation," I say to Betty. "Sydney doesn't have disability access either. It's disheartening! It's outrageous!"

"Well, it's a young population," Betty counters.

"There are old people here!"

"There are old people everywhere, but I'm not talking about people. I'm talking about the population. That's different."

I hang up angry and tell Ernest about the conversation.

"It was a young country," Ernest says, smiling. "A hundred and fifty years ago."

I call my host in Sydney. "We have the same baby boom problem that America has," she says. "But our government is not doing anything about it. They say it will be too expensive."

I call Betty back immediately and point-prove. I'll be damned if I won't be the "top-dog" sociologist, the position I've always held vis-à-vis Betty.

"It's all political," she says.

"It's social and cultural and economic," I counter.

We get into an argument about how politics and culture intersect. I am seething. Do I think this will be our last conversation? Do I want it to be our last conversation? Do I want this to be over? What would be over? My feelings of responsibility? My unfinished book? Who is this woman? Do I even know her?

Saturday, March 19

If Betty is not who she was, who is dying?

Monday, March 21

The sunset seen from our Elizabeth Avenue apartment is spectacular!

Packing up is easy.

Late dinner at "our" fantabulous pan-Asian restaurant is easy.

Leaving Australia is easy.

Friday, March 24
Papeete, Tahiti

Dear Betty,

There's no way to phone from here or to mail a letter, so I'll write this to you in my Daybook.

Remember how excited I was about going to Tahiti? And how thrilled you were for me? Well . . .

After Ernest drove the Peugeot (all instructions and road signage in French) from the airport to downtown Papeete (sans map), lugged (no porter) the luggage from its insides (WARNING: Leave Nothing in Your Car! Not even in your locked boot), and carted said luggage (no trolley) to the slamming-door elevator to our second-floor corner room at the Mandarin Hotel, and after we had dispensed all of our Tahitian coins into the air-conditioning unit, leaving us none for purchasing bottled water, and after the roosters in our side yard had pulled an all-nighter, their cock-a-doodle dos resounding off the tin exterior walls, and after Ernest had to get up at 5:30 a.m. to move the car before it got towed, and after one of his feet was as big as two and his stomach felt quite queasy, we decided to make the Mandarin Hotel a one-night stand.

Because none of the Papeete streets allow parking and we were shooed off the Tourist Bureau lot, we drove to the one place we knew we could park—the airport. A lovely (English speaking!) woman at Hertz Rental Car, the only kiosk open in the airport, negotiated a room for us at the Sofitel about half an hour's drive up (down?) the coast. The Sofitel did allow parking.

Our large beachfront room is clean, quiet, and supplied with bottled water. From our balcony we see lush tropical plantings around an Olympic-sized pool, a small crescent-shaped sandy beach, a saltwater lagoon majestic in turquoise, green, and blue, the volcanic island Mooréa, and above all of this sky-blue pink and sky-blue blue and dragon clouds. I have never seen a more beautiful view.

Ernest stayed in bed with food poisoning. I read, slept, swam, took a (French-speaking) tour bus to the Gauguin Museum, but it was closed. I visited the highly advertised and highly guarded Tahiti "Black Pearl Market." It is not a marketplace at all but a narrow inside space with three walk-up floors. Large, dark, round, unblemished pearls are on the top floor, some selling for four thousand dollars—per pearl! I was homesick for my white ones. Thankfully, we leave for home tonight. Talk to you soon.

Cheers, l

Sunday, March 26

> To: Maisie
> From: richardson
> Subject: Home again
>
> hi—we're exhausted, of course. . . . tahiti was something of a
> nightmare—ernest had turista, our plane was 9 hours late, we waited
> all night in an un-air-conditioned, un-serviced (no drinking water)
> airport, we missed our connections—it took 44 hours to get home!!!
> wanted to let you know we are here. . . . I assume Kingsley has
> sent my honorarium. . . . off to bed for me. (347 e-mails on my screen
> here!!)
>
> g'day, I

"Hi, Betty. We're home." I leave the message on Penny's answering
machine. Winter has passed, and I am trying to get my mind around
Betty's not having died.

Monday, March 27

While Ernest is at the foot doctor, I take stock of Betty's situation. She
is taking Xanax and ten other medications. Sometimes she can walk
across the room in her walker. She spends "half her time sleeping, and
the other half not being able to get the words out of her mouth." She
has incessant coughing, digestive problems, and hives. She has screaming
pain from her lower back that does not subside with muscle relaxants or
lying on the foam-core mattress that Penny bought. Penny takes her to
doctor appointments, Mike takes her to the casino, and Jack takes her
for rides in the golf cart. She's sick but she has a daughter, son-in-law,
and grandson who take care of her.

I don't know if I will.

Tuesday, March 28

"I'm complacent about the whole *subject*," Betty says, alluding to her
dying. "It should bother me, but it doesn't. I can't talk about it though
without jumping into someone else's shoes, trying to take care of them."

"Hospice can talk about the subject," I say.

Silence.

"You're not ready to go, are you?"

"I don't understand it, but no, I guess I am not. I've gone over some hump. I'm not frantic and crazy fighting it."

"Do you remember what my Aunt Ceil used to say?" Aunt Ceil said that every day she found something in life that gave her pleasure, even though she had congestive heart failure and twice-weekly blood transfusions for leukemia.

"I think of your Aunt Ceil every day," Betty says. "But it's not one little thing that gives me pleasure, it's lots of little things that I wouldn't even have noticed before that give me pleasure. Life is basic. Nature trumps culture."

Wednesday, March 29

Today's the day to reclaim Mimi-the-cat from her vacation in the country visiting with four other cats. When we come in, Mimi is sitting on "her" cushion at the top of the stairs, ears back, the whites of her eyes showing. We put her into her carrying case, pack her things, and put her and them into the car. She wails for the first forty minutes. "We'll just have to get her a kitten," I say. When we turn onto Dublin-Granville Road, she stops her caterwauling. When we turn down Evening Street, she begins to purr. When we turn into our driveway, her purr is a roar. Inside the house she snuggles into my lap. "I guess Mimi likes being 'Only Cat,'" I say. She knows her place.

Thursday, March 30

"From being here at Penny's, I've learned that I really didn't know much about people," Betty tells me. "The people here are so ordinary, I'm bored. I don't know how they get through life. I'd be sleeping like Rip Van Winkle."

For as long as I've known Betty, she's been afraid of being "ordinary," although I've never quite known what she means by *ordinary*. She thought her concert-pianist mother was ordinary and her accountant father was not. I ask her about her father now.

"My father wasn't ordinary because he had an extraordinary ability to love and laugh," she says.

But everything I've heard about Penny and Mike's friends and family suggests that they are loving and full of laughter.

"You often found it boring in Kent too," I say.

"In Kent there's always the chance that I can get out for lunch and that people might come to visit."

"In Delaware there's always the chance Mike will take you to the casino."

"Now that's not boring."

"You get lots of phone calls there too," I say. Does she think her callers are ordinary?

"Ellyn. Bless her. Every third day like clockwork. She sent me our high school newsletter. Big spread on Phillip Roth."

"Bonnie?"

"Bonnie told me she thinks I'm valiant."

"Pam?"

"Dear Pam. She sent me a six-page list of people who could take care of me in Kent."

"David?"

"David's lovely. He's taking care of my Kent house, watering my plants, picking up the flyers."

"Alfred?"

"He always has a joke for me."

"Rhonda?"

"Ha! Forget her. All she does is talk about herself."

What about me? I wonder. Am I ordinary? I don't ask.

Friday, March 31

It's a common, *ordinary* story—the bedside reconciliation between the living and dying—but that is not the reconciliation story I am struggling with now. Rather, I am unwillingly immersed in trying to reconcile my understanding of Betty, myself, and our friendship with what I am learning through the writing of the Daybook about her, me, and the friendship.

There's so little I have known about the deeper, less-transparent Betty. Our conversation about *ordinary*, though, has forced me into that uncharted terrain. Thinking about this is emotional and intellectual work. I take a deep breath and enter Betty's "philosophy of life."

Betty does not see herself as a causal actor in her own life, and therefore she does not own responsibility for her feelings. If she feels bored, it must be the fault of the people around her—they are *ordinary*. *Ordinary* is code, a way of externalizing "I'm bored."

Sometimes I can only understand something by looking at its opposite. So I ask myself, *When is Betty not bored?*

Betty's not bored when she is the center of attention, when friends bring her things, tell her jokes, and listen to her problems, when doctors ask about "each of her body parts and listen to her answers," and when her father "loved everything she did." But in Delaware she's not, as she had hoped, "the stillness around which everything circulates."

And Betty is not bored when a person, place, or thing ignites her imagination, feeds her fantasies. Those fantasies are stoked by *chance*. Talking to strangers on trains, truck stops, sidewalk smoking pits is not boring: there's always the chance that something *un*-ordinary might happen. Playing the slots, betting on the horses, pooling on the lottery is not boring: there's always the chance of hitting the jackpot. Being home in Kent with her car in the driveway is not boring: there's always the chance that someone will stop by or she'll be able to drive around the corner for a Coke at Burger King. How dismal these last months must have been for her without a chance of escaping in reality or in fantasy.

In some ways Betty and I are opposites. I believe I have some control over what I think and do, if not the outcome. I find games of chance boring, but there is almost nothing I think of as ordinary, except in a positive sense—an ordinary day, an uneventful plane ride, a commonplace walk to the grocery. And I don't like fantasy—in movies, books, or my psyche.

When I was in my thirties and dealing with a challenging family situation, I didn't want to talk about anything to anyone for fear that I'd talk about everything. I sought self-centered friends because they took the conversational burden off me. But Betty was *the* friend I could talk to. We were conversational partners—taking turns being self-centered. My self-centeredness was needier and more intense than Betty's, as I had more pressing strife in my life than she did in hers. I spilled out my woes, fears, and anxieties. She never cut me off. She never said, "Enough already, Laurel. Enough." I don't know how I would have gotten through those dark years without her.

So now the tables are turned.

It's okay by me for Betty to be the center.

It's her turn.

So is our friendship extraordinary or just ordinary?

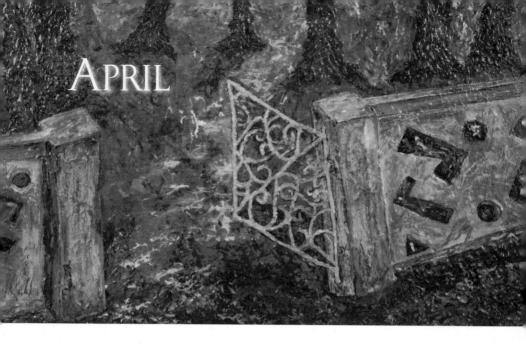

APRIL

Saturday, April 1

"What's that noise?" I hearing a click-clicking I can't identity over the phone.

"It's the parakeet," Betty says.

"Parakeet? When did you get that?"

"It's Jack's. They think it'll keep me company. There's two of them."

I don't like parakeets or their dumb tricks, but I don't say anything.

"Quiet!" she yells.

"So how're you?"

"It's been a bad morning. Bad week."

"How come?"

"Benign neglect. These are very, very busy people. Always doing. I think Penny's way of avoiding thinking about me is by doing, doing, doing. Next week she'll be taking FEMA classes, unless there is some disaster."

We chuckle.

"Wasn't it April first when you had your own little disaster driving home in the dark from Trumball Campus?" I say.

"Yeah. All around the road were carcasses and then I hit a deer," Betty says.

"You weren't injured but the Sable's front end was," I continue. "Your CB radio didn't work but a stranger, a woman, stopped and called Triple A."

"You don't forget anything, do you, Laurel?"

When I was a preschooler, my father began training my memory. Mother was to tell me the grocery list, adding items as they occurred to her. It was my responsibility to make sure all items were purchased when she and I went to the store. If I forgot something, the whole family "suffered." Indelibly writ upon my little soul was the idea that remembering things is a way of acting responsibly, morally.

"Faces," I say. "Can't ever remember a face. But voices, conversations, spoken words . . ."

Sunday, April 2

"Herds of elephants," Betty says. "Rogue elephants with diamond collars invade my dreams. Elephant bones surround the phone poles."

Tuesday, April 4

"How're you doin'?" I ask.

"Not so—*cough*—good. *Cough cough.* The doctor says I'm to be in the wheelchair all the time."

"Sorry," I say. "Ernest's restricted now too because of his plantar fasciitis."

Long pause.

"*Cough cough.* The kids brought me pots of yellow dahlias."

"Dahlias?"

Long pause.

"I watched the sunset last night," she says.

Long pause.

"Hey, I have a joke for you," I say. "My water aerobics teacher told it to the class. Two ninety-year-olds had dated for about six months when the man asks the woman, 'Can we be more intimate?' She says, 'You mean have sex,' and he says, 'Yes.' After the event, the man says to himself, *If I had known she was a virgin, I would have been gentler.* The woman says to herself, *If I had known he could get it up, I would have taken off my panty hose.*"

Betty laughs.

Has it come to this? Me telling Betty jokes so I'll have something to say?

"I'm going to Artiscape tomorrow," I say. I am still tired. "I've signed up for seven workshops on making paper and books. Talk to you when I get back."

"You bet."

I am very lonely.

Monday, April 10

I am back from Artiscape even more tired. I have spent the weekend making fancy papers, and learning collage, printing, and pop-up techniques. In the pop-up book class I succeeded in making only three messy signatures instead of the assigned neat four. Admiring a perfectly squared four-signature book, the instructor said, "It's the best in the class. What I had in mind." Of my work she said, "Oh, you're making art."

Last year I loved Artiscape, but this year I am too tired and judgmental about my art and the droves of big-bottomed, serious, and "ordinary" women crafters. They all came with friends. Another place where I do not belong.

"The Artiscape women like to craft the way Penny does," I tell Betty on the phone. "I don't have much in common with them."

I feel stupid bringing Penny into this. I am trying too hard to stay in Betty's world, trying to make my world relevant to hers, and maybe trying to elicit her sympathy.

"My dear son Josh has gone to the career counselor three times now," I say. I am pleased about this. "But he still doesn't have a car. He can't afford to repair his, and he can't find one he can afford to buy."

Betty loves Josh. Maybe she will sell him her car. I certainly can't ask her.

While Betty and I are talking, Jack comes home from school, walks through her apartment, and leaves. Penny comes home from work, greets Betty, and leaves to say hello to Jack. Mike comes in with Betty's dinner, about which she says, "Add some salt." Each time someone comes into her apartment I say, "I'll call back later," but she wants me to remain on the phone.

"I'm coming back to Kent on May fifth," Betty announces. "But I don't think I'll be able to manage back home." She then tells me a story I've heard several times before.

"My first memory," she says, "was seeing my grandfather laid out in a wooden box in our living room. He had been tall, thin, with silver hair and bright blue eyes. Although he was a junk man, everyone said that he had more dignity than anyone. That it should happen to him . . . that he should die on the toilet . . . tsk-tsk."

Betty takes after her grandfather. She too is thin, silver-haired, and blue-eyed.

"I fell off the toilet Friday," she says. "The first image that came to my mind was my grandfather in that wooden box."

"Did you get hurt?"

"Nothing broken, but I couldn't get up. No one was home. I didn't have the phone or pager with me."

"Bruises?"

"Not really. Penny had told me that if I knew I was going to fall, I should just relax into it. So I did."

"So how'd it happen?"

"I was reading a newspaper and leaning forward, and I lost my balance, and then I was on the floor."

"I'm so sorry."

"My dignity was hurt the most. After a long time I managed to get up somehow and got back into bed. I was shaking the rest of the day. I don't know how I can go home to Kent."

"Oh, Betty."

"I want to spend the summer in Kent."

I am surprised that she envisions herself living through the summer.

"I plan to see you in May or June wherever you are," I say.

"That will be very nice. Oh, and I'm getting $2000 back from Uncle Sam. I'm going to buy a Serta bed to help my back. I need to find out how easy it will be to disassemble it so I can move it back to Penny's next winter."

I think about my cousin Katie and the spending spree she went on for durable goods—new glasses, a walker, wheels—the month before she died of cancer.

Wednesday, April 12

"Hi, Betty. Happy Passover."

"Six thousand years of tradition and here it has stopped," Betty replies. She still feels guilty that she did not raise Penny Jewish.

"Someone else will carry on the tradition," I say. "That's how it's always been."

"Yeah." She doesn't sound convinced. She has given her aide, Norma, the recipe for making the Passover *tzimmes*—sweet potato, meat, dried onions, prunes—and I can hear Norma in the background asking, "What do you call *this*?"

"It's a warm sunny day here," I say. "Not the cruelest month at all."

"As we speak, Mike is plowing the garden plot."

"Can you get out in your wheelchair?"

"Sure, I'll hitch up the horses."

"Still looking for that cowboy, huh?"

"No white horses in sight."

"But hey, Cowgirl, you've recovered from your fall."

"Not psychologically. I am still disturbed by that image of my grandfather."

"I remember when you first told me that story," I say.

"I remember where I told it to you. We were on the cement steps of your Kenworth house by the river . . ."

". . . probably watching the children play on the lawn. . . . That was a long time ago."

"I don't remember why I told you that story," she says.

"I don't either. Maybe we were talking about death . . ."

". . . or childhood . . ."

". . . or our first memories . . ."

". . . or our grandfathers."

"Yes. I think that was it," I say. "Both of our first memories are of our grandfathers.

"And now we've become them," she says, but doesn't laugh.

Friday, April 14

I sleep in and wake up feeling punk, even though the day is bright and warm. I eat my kasha cereal, read the paper, talk to my son Ben. After lunch I read Ernest my Daybook entry about my feelings at Artiscape. He is rolling his injured foot on a rubber ball.

"What you should be doing is writing your Daybook," he says. "This is where your energy should be going. Writing is your métier. You shouldn't be going off to art retreats and losing your focus."

He has clarity about so much.

"I associate all my writing with being a sociologist, a professor," I say. "It's more complex for me than it has been for you." When Ernest was fifty-two—fifteen years ago—he retired from the Department of English at The Ohio State University, and he has never looked back. After retiring, he continued writing fiction and cowrote our memoir, *Travels With Ernest*. He polished up his clarinet and three saxes and formed the South Street Jazz Band. Now he no longer plans to write and has disbanded the jazz band. He's morphed into a painter of large-scale acrylics.

I ponder his opinion and try to accept his compliment. I like to write. Why do I think I should stop? Why can't I disassociate my writing from my academic career?

Saturday, April 15

I'm walking around the neighborhood when I reach Betty in her apartment on my cell phone.

"I'm exhausted but in a good kind of way," she says. "Penny's taken me to the Serta bed store. The bed's terrific, but it costs $2000."

"So what?" I say. "You've got the $2000 from Uncle Sam." This is a typical conversational exchange. A dance. Betty forgets what she had previously told me and I call her on it.

"The salesclerk also says it's too cumbersome and heavy to take in a truck."

My cue to "problem solve." Mike and Penny are strong. Buy the bed in Kent. Have it delivered. Hire someone to assemble it. Hire someone to disassemble it, and so on, ad nauseam. Typical steps in our dance.

"No one believes I'm going home," Betty asserts. "The more they say I am not, the more I am determined to do so."

"You go on May fifth."

"May sixth." Another dance step. "I need to convince Penny that she doesn't have to come back to Kent every time I get sick there. I've told her I don't want done to me what they did to me in October."

"They took you to the hospital and resuscitated you in October, and they did that in Delaware too." She has been in the hospital five times since she arrived in Delaware.

"I don't remember."

"If you don't want to be resuscitated, then you can't go to the hospital. If you go to the hospital, they'll do it." I feel as if I am pushing her to accept her dying. I have accepted it. At least I think I have. More dancing.

"I've proved the doctor wrong. Two years ago he said I would be dead this April. He was wrong."

I draw in my breath. We're only halfway though the month of April, but I don't argue with her, take that dance step. Instead, I say, "That's pretty awful to give someone a death date."

"He was gentle about it. And I pushed him."

Another one of Betty's secrets? Am I glad or miffed that she kept the doctor's prognosis from me? Glad. I'm glad.

Pas de deux.

"I'll not go to the hospital unless it becomes impossible not to," Betty says.

"What do you mean?"

"Too hard on Penny, Mike, and Jack."

"You mean while you're in Delaware?"

The pause is so long that I realize Betty means Kent, Ohio, too. She's good at finessing.

"I've told Penny, I've lived my life," Betty says. "It's over. Whatever's left is gravy."

Betty loves gravy.

Tuesday, April 18

"How're you?" I ask Betty. I am walking the neighborhood again on a lovely spring day. Every fruit tree is in blossom.

We chat about the old pain in her back and the new pain in her gums, the old pain in her stomach and the new pain in her neck, and then she says, "I can't *hear* you."

"I can't hear you either. . . . I'll talk to you later."

I think she says, "You bet."

Our connection was so much better when I was in Australia.

Wednesday, April 19

I don't like Betty.

Saturday, April 22

I've been cogitating on not liking Betty for days. I don't want to phone her and I don't want to write in this Daybook. But I will.

Maybe I have the "Truman Capote syndrome." Capote wanted his "subject," Perry Smith, to die so he could finish his book, *In Cold Blood*.

I am forlorn.

When someone has a long illness, bit by bit you lose what you had in common. The mourning process, the experience of loss after loss, goes on while the person is still alive. After a while, if the person does not die, there is little of the relationship left. There's little left to talk about other than the person's illness, pains, and the inevitability that lies ahead. You're worn out from the constant grief work. What was once a voluntary act—a phone call, a visit, a card—becomes obligatory. You never can do enough. You can never make it all right. You might even wish the person dead already.

Am I willing to let these words stand?

I don't have the deep sadness that propelled me into keeping this Daybook. And I don't have the anger I had when Betty decided against hospice.

What I feel now is disgust. Betty brought her lung problems upon herself by refusing to give up smoking. Then, a few months ago, long after it was too late, she finally gave it up. Doing so has prolonged her pain and suffering and the pain and suffering of those around her as they participate in her deterioration. She's always craved attention. Now she has it—in spades!

Oh, Betty! I think you've become the person you've hated all your life—your mother. You are doing your dying the way she did hers. She refused to submit, demanded care and attention, reveled in being center stage as though reliving the pinnacle of her life, her piano concert at Carnegie Hall. Your father, her eternal fan, hastened to her every beck and call. What high point might you be reliving? Who responds to your beck and call?

We've been friends for thirty-five years and I know so little about you.

Monday, April 24

For years I have advised my students to write down their unbearably embarrassing feelings about people they are studying. By writing these feelings down, the feelings lose their hold on you. I guess this is good advice. My feeling of disgust no longer dominates.

I call Betty and ask her if she remembers our Carole Little outfits. She does. And does she remember where we bought them? She does. In Washington at Saks. And does she still have the outfit? She does, and she still wears it.

We have a benign shopping history that I can retrieve and relive.

"Did I tell you I was altering a Nancy Drew book for the Qualitative Inquiry Conference?"

"Nancy Drew was never one of my favorites," Betty says.

Normally I would respond to this conversational put-down defensively, but I don't now.

"She sure was mine." I say, without edginess.

"I still remember you telling me that Jo in *Little Women* was not your role model," Betty says, in a neutral tone. "I still can't figure that out. Jo was a tomboy. Independent. She liked her freedom."

I don't challenge Betty. I don't start my response with the obliquely dismissive "but."

Instead I say, "I liked Nancy Drew best because she had a red roadster, a boyfriend, a criminal lawyer father, no mother. And she could solve problems." My voice stays even.

"She was filthy rich!" Betty says with disgust.

"And Jo was poor."

"It isn't fair—rich people have all the advantages."

Would you rather still be poor? I almost ask, but don't. Betty grew up poor. I did not.

"This has been interesting," she says.

"Someone" has put "something weird" on her bed tray.

"Talk to you later," I say.

"You bet."

We've had this conversation about books many times over the years. Now I realize its value in our friendship. How easily we deflect our profound differences onto our differences over storybook heroines.

Tuesday, April 25

I am shopping at Polaris, a megamall surrounded by big box stores. I punch NPR on my car radio. Terry Gross is in the middle of an interview with the psychologist Dan Gottlieb. She asks him a very gross question, something like "while you were supposed to be dead—so few live with quadriplegia into their fifties—so while you were supposed to be dead, other people who were supposed to stay on in your life left —your ex-wife left, your sister died of a brain tumor—I mean people seemed to be healthy, and then they're gone. So how do you feel about this?" This is what she asked, more or less. A long silence ensued. I thought maybe Gottlieb's quadriplegia affected his speech generally. Then he said, "I don't know how to respond to that." Another long pause. Then he said something like, "We wouldn't have life without death. We wouldn't understand it. The closer I come to death, the more precious the daytime is and the nighttime is and the more grateful I feel. The immanence of death makes life more alive."

As I drive across Polaris Parkway with the green light, a black beaten-up car runs the red light and makes a left turn into my lane. I veer, and the black car goes speeding on its way. Today is not my day to be rendered a quadriplegic. Nor my day to die.

I better understand Betty's desire to stay alive. There must be something addictive to experiencing the end of life. As one strips away the extraneous from one's life, narrows one's life to the immediate and the sensory, those experiences must grow in intensity. Sweets must seem sweeter, sunshine sunnier, bluebirds bluer.

Wednesday, April 26

"I've had a great week," Betty says. "Mike took me for a ride out into the country. It was gorgeous. Everything was in bloom. We went to the casino and I won $360."

"I don't know how you do it," I say. "You always play the slots and you always win. What's your secret?"

"You keep playing a winning machine," she says.

"Yeah. Uh-huh. Okay, Betty. I've never had a winning machine."

"I go home to Kent in ten days," Betty says. "But I'm afraid I'll be in the hospital and won't be able to make the trip."

I hear someone come into Betty's apartment. It sounds like Penny. "Is that Penny?"

"It's Jack. . . . I've told you not to do that, Jack. Get out of here!"

"What happening?"

"He jumped up behind my wheelchair. . . . Get! Get out of here! Now!"

Thursday, April 27

It was probably twelve years ago on a surprisingly warm April day like this one that Betty and I reclined on the blue lawn chaises in my backyard by the sundial. Etched around the sundial's metal face is the saying "Grow old with me, the best it yet to be." We were drinking iced tea and Betty was smoking. After putting her butts out on the ground, she lined them up on the sundial's base. I had carefully planned an intervention. "Betty," I said. "It's your life to do with as you please. But I need to tell you how angry and sad it makes me that you're destroying your health and shortening your life. Quit smoking for my sake, if not for yours." We almost stopped being friends forever.

Betty never again came to my house.

Saturday, April 29

I am at an art retreat in Laurel Lodge at Lake Hope with eleven other women, including two dear friends, Julie and Merry. We are so isolated that nobody's cell phone works. Our homes are two hours and two centuries away. We have set ourselves up to work outside on picnic tables. The sun warms our hands and a slight breeze carries the scent of spring green.

"Do you ever just feel happy?" Merry asks.

"I do," I say. "I am."

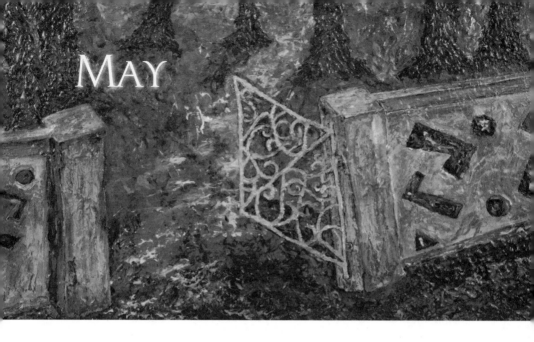

MAY

Monday, May 1

"Betty, I'll be gone for five days to the Qualitative Inquiry Conference," I say.

"Have a good time," she says. She sounds weak.

Sunday, May 7

At the Qualitative Inquiry Conference I present my new altered book work on Nancy Drew, serve on an old-timers' panel, and attend four sessions about loss, grief, and mourning. I sleep a lot.

"Betty's in the hospital in Delaware," Ernest tells me as we drive home from the Columbus airport. He looks rested. "Ellyn called to tell you. I like her."

"She's great," I agree. "She's a therapist, you know, and she'll be a major support for me when Betty dies."

Once home I go through my e-mail and snail mail—still no honorarium from Dean Kingsley. I decide to let it go. After calling my children, sister, and brother, I go for a walk and eat my dinner. When I finally phone the hospital, it takes nine calls to reach Betty.

"I dunno nothin'," says the first answerer.

"She's not here no more," says the second.

"I will transfer you to admissions," says the third.

"There was someone in this room. She's not here now. I'll ask the nurse to help. I can't figure out how to use the call button . . . sorry. . . . Can you figure it out, Hon? No, . . . sorry." This was the fourth's valiant attempt. She was a patient.

"She is in room 420A. I'll transfer you," says the fifth.

"Why is the phone ringing here at the front desk? Doesn't the phone pick up in 420A?" Elevator bells in the background. Laughter. Chatter. "She's not here." The sixth was a nurse.

"How do you spell that name? *How?* I can't transfer you. . . . No. . . . What? No, I don't know the hospital's main phone number. . . . No. . . . I don't know how to find that number." The seventh was the patient information desk.

"I jes' start workin' here. . . . No, I dunno know the name of the hospital," says the eighth, a kind-sounding aide who happened to be passing by a ringing phone.

"Hello . . . *cough.*" At last, Betty's gravelly voice.

"Hi," I say. "It's near impossible to get into this hospital by phone. How'd you manage to get your whole body in?"

Betty laughs. "I got pneumonia. That's how."

"Looks like the man on the white horse you've wanted to rescue you all these years has morphed into the man in the white scrubs."

She laughs.

"How long have you been there?"

"Since the day you left. They've moved me around to a lot of different rooms. Now I'm in the 'penthouse.' A room so huge that the bathroom is a room away. Only one picture on the wall, and that's gray and next to the television, which is behind a pole."

"Do you have a view?"

"It's a crappy day."

"I'm so sorry you've had to miss the May fourth events in Kent."

May 4 is the most significant day in Betty's adult life.

Our stories are always partial. Stories always fall short. Some stories are too hard to tell, so we make up ones we can live with. When truths become too slippery, we look for other ones to hold onto. I do not know the official story or the unofficial stories of May 4, but I will tell the story in a way that I think Betty could live with, although not totally endorse, because in my telling I will be who I am. I will fail to lay blame.

On May 4, 1970, the Ohio National Guard fired on Kent State University students, leaving four of them dead and nine wounded. Betty taught at the Kent State's Trumball Campus but lived walking distance from the main one. She was active in university politics and had directed its first Women's Project. She was on the main campus May 4.

On Friday evening, May 1, students, many inebriated, rallied against the invasion of Cambodia. They broke windows in downtown Kent, overturned cars, and threw rocks at the police. When rumors of a radical plot circulated, the mayor called the governor, who called out the Ohio National Guard. The police closed the bars and teargassed hundreds of people, herding them to the dorms. By 2:30 a.m. the town was as quiet as it always had been.

On May 2 some students cleaned up the downtown, while others threatened the merchants with more violence. The university got an injunction against further rallies and leafleted it widely around campus. Just after 8:00 p.m., with more than a thousand people surrounding the Army Reserve training center, the building was set on fire. Unable to extinguish the fire because demonstrators cut and punctured their fire hoses, the firemen departed, letting the building burn to the ground. No one was hurt. By midnight the National Guard cleared the campus, again herding demonstrators into the dorms.

May 3 began in calm, but later crowds gathered on campus. They were read the Riot Act but they failed to disperse. At 9:00 p.m. tear gas was fired, and the crowd moved downtown, blocking traffic. At 11:00 p.m. the Riot Act was read downtown to no effect. Tear gas was fired. Guardsmen and demonstrators scuffled, and many were injured.

Classes resumed on Monday, May 4. Two thousand people gathered in the commons area. Many—but not all, especially the commuters—knew the rally had been banned. Curses, rock throwing, and general baiting answered the guardsmen's calls to disperse. Tear gas was set off shortly after noon, but the wind swept it away from the demonstrators. Guardsmen moved forward with fixed bayonets, moving the crowd over the crest of Taylor Hill to an athletic field that was surrounded by a fence on three sides. Demonstrators threw curses and rocks. Guardsman threw tear gas again and backed up. Two thousand demonstrators closed in on them, some as close as twenty yards. Over the crest, twenty-eight guardsmen fired sixty-one to sixty-seven shots in thirteen seconds. Four students were dead, nine wounded.

Betty was with a crowd of people on the slope, behind the burned-out building, when the shots were fired. Even those near her who had been in Vietnam thought they were hearing firecrackers. The news that bullets had been fired passed to the crowd on the slope. Betty left campus before the first ambulance arrived.

Each year May 4 is commemorated at Kent State University with several days of speeches, folksinging, students' issues, and a candlelight vigil. Several thousand come to confirm their commitments to peace and justice. Betty's friends who currently or previously lived in Kent take part in these public events and in private ones. One year Betty gave a speech describing the rise and fall of the Women's Project at Kent State. She didn't stint on her criticism of the university's administration. It was a courageous talk.

In 1977, following years of legal battles, Kent State won the right to build a gymnasium on the ground where the deaths had occurred. Betty's picture was in the paper. She was in her raincoat and rain hat, on a bended knee, head lowered like a baby lamb, hand covering her eyes, her tears. She told me she was protecting a tree. She lost. The tree was bulldozed, the gymnasium was built. Power trumps powerlessness.

Now I ask her on the phone, "How does it feel to have missed the May fourth commemorations? The first time you've missed them, right?"

"The truth of the matter," she says, sighing, "is that I feel so disconnected from everything now that I don't feel anything."

Monday, May 8

I dream I have three pieces of luggage. One, a square green box in which

I have put all my leftovers without securing the lid, I put on the roof of a stranger's car. The box gets lost.

Am I trying to get rid of everything in my life that is "left over"?

This is the happiest time of my life. Yet I wish I were young, again.

Tuesday, May 9

"Hi, Betty," I say. "I'm walking my path at the club. Any news?"

"The morning doctor says I'm 'bad' and the afternoon doctor says I'm 'good.' What do I know? Both of them say the mucous plug is not dissolving, but the pneumonia is improving. I'm so sick of being sick."

"You've been saying that for the last six years," I say.

We laugh. But I don't think it's very funny. I am bored with her "sick of being sick."

"I want you to rewrite my obituary," she says. "Tell my story. I've done more in my life than the measly three paragraphs we wrote in October. Tell them I was there at May fourth. Tell them I fought for women's rights at Kent State University. Tell them I knocked on doors to find feminist faculty. Tell them."

Wednesday, May 10

"What's up?" I ask.

"Radishes," Betty answers. She's back in her apartment at Penny's. "Penny spent the entire day pulling up radishes."

We discuss how I might manage a visit to Betty. No commercial planes fly into the entire state of Delaware. I'll have to fly to Baltimore and then either rent a car and drive some two hours through city traffic, over the Annapolis Bridge onto country back lanes, or take a taxicab for six hundred dollars round trip.

Thursday, May 11

My birthday will be July 15, and as it approaches I become more discomfited by my uncertainty about what I want to do to mark it or even if I want to mark it. Maybe all I want to do is hide until it is over. But as I think and write about Betty's illness and how all of our days are numbered, I make a different decision. From this moment on, I designate this entire year as my Birth Celebration, the way arts communities do for famous artists and musicians. My audacity tickles me.

Today, then, is the first of the many days of my Birth Celebration. I meet with my dear friend Marilyn. We've been friends for a quarter century. For the past decade we've met a couple times a year at the Winds Café in Yellow Springs, a site of peace, hippieness, and beauty, midway between our two home cities. Marilyn is a few years older than I am. She's been a beacon to me, a model of how to move gracefully into each new stage of life, how to look out the window at the grass and accept that that is enough, and how to endure physical challenges. A few years back Marilyn decided to volunteer at hospice because she wanted to know more about that stage of life.

"My friend Betty has refused to go into hospice," I tell Marilyn, as I settle into my lunch of organic brown rice, tofu, and raw cashews. "She seems to be on a teeter-totter. Every time her breathing gets worse she goes to the hospital and they treat her. Then she goes home for a bit, and then she's back in the hospital. During the past six months she's spent half her time in the hospital. Is this ordinary?"

"What do you mean?" Marilyn asks.

"Is this a common way for people to approach death?"

Marilyn's answer is simple and straightforward. "She's not ready to die."

"She says she is," I reply. "She says she's 'let go.'"

"She doesn't believe *she* is dying. She's not ready to let go of . . .," Marilyn touches her hand to her heart, ". . . to let go of her desire to be in this world."

I make a puzzled face.

"Did I tell you about when I almost died?" Marilyn asks.

"Tell me again."

"I went to the doctor's for a routine check," she begins, "when he discovered something that alarmed him. He immediately checked me into the hospital. A cardiologist arrived and rechecked me. It seems I was throwing blood clots and that any one of them could have gone to my lungs or my brain and killed me—or worse. The chances of my living through the night were not good. I said good-bye to my husband and to my best friend, Joan. Joan said, 'I'm not ready for you to leave me,' and I said, 'You may not have a choice.'

"I was alone in my room at 9 p.m. I brought into my mind's eye each of my children and grandchildren, and one by one I sent them gratitude for being in my life and let them know I was able to let them go. I thought about all the people who had been important to me—you were one of them, Laurel—"

"Thanks."

"—and I looked at each one in my mind and thanked them and let them go. By 3:30 in the morning I had said good-bye to everyone, and I fell asleep. I woke up at 9 a.m. and said to myself, 'I guess I am still alive. That's nice.'"

We sit in silence for a bit, and then order two chocolate mousses.

We leave the café in a light sprinkling of rain. Warmth rises from the sidewalk.

"I've become so sensuous lately," I say to Marilyn. "So much more aware of the sensuousness of my everyday world. Tastes and textures, like brown rice, the smell of the lilacs that line my driveway, the greening of grass, the comfort of these raindrops on my hair, the warmth rising from the sidewalk."

We walk along together.

Friday, May 12

When did this happen? Friends and family routinely asking me, "How's Betty?"

Sunday, May 14

Merry and I are eating lunch on her new deck, and she asks me about my time at the Qualitative Inquiry Conference.

"It was a life-affirming conference," I say. "People from all the over the world and in many different disciplines know my work. I felt appreciated, loved, and beloved."

"So you can stop doing the work now," Merry says.

"Quite the opposite," I say. "There are audiences for my work, and I love doing it—I love to write. I've been telling myself I have to stop, and now I realize I don't. Retirement does not mean giving up that which gives me and others pleasure." My certainty surprises me.

"What's more," I continue, "I have found a *place* where I belong—a community of international, interdisciplinary, arts and sciences, theory and practice inscribers and performers." I did say all of that, maybe in a different order, but I did say all of that because I had surprised myself even more by the breadth and depth of the world to which I felt personally connected.

"Very life-affirming," Merry agrees.

"Yes. And life-reaffirming," I like finding the right word. *Reaffirming*. My chosen way of being in the world is not over. "And you know what?"

"What?"

"I'm eager to begin another book, a book focused on my life rather than Betty's."

A nightmare I'd had in Melbourne reenters my mind. In the nightmare I was facilitating a writing workshop with elderly people. What was it I asked them to do? Ah, yes: *Tell about something in their lives that mattered to them.*

So what matters to *me*?

Monday, May 15

I finish what I start, an edict I cross-stitched twenty years ago when working on another book, is on my wall in front of my computer, staring me in my face. When I finished that book, I bought myself a strand of pearls. Pearls bring "good luck and a long life," the saleswoman said.

Maybe I don't have to finish what I start.

Finish has become a troublesome word for me of late. I get a lot "done," but I don't "finish" many things. In the basement family room there's a pile of children's books and toys on the floor in the corner, unsorted. In the back of the basement, three file cabinets are partially divested of syllabi, reprints, and articles, but the collecting together of my "Collected Works" has not happened. Some of those works gather dust on top of the files, while others look like they have been trashed in a box too near Mimi's litter box. Two garbage bags of clothes for the

Kidney Foundation stand like sentinels over two boxes of household goods, also for the Kidney Foundation, but I haven't called to have them picked up. My basement bookcases are crammed to overflowing with books I will never read again but have not packed into boxes for the Friends of the Library. My mind quickly scans my other spaces—study, studio, kitchen, bathrooms, bedroom, closets. Way too much stuff. But do I want to spend my time "decluttering?" Isn't that what kids are supposed to do after you die? Get rid of your stuff?

Am I decluttering my mind now of Betty's life? Getting ready to focus on mine?

Tuesday, May 16

With gusto I begin decluttering my shoes. I am determined not only to get something *done* about my shoes but also to *finish* the project. Change the behavior and the attitude will follow. That's a sociological research finding I can apply to my life! If I declutter my shoes, surely my mind will follow.

Why *shoes* now?

It's Betty again. For me, Betty and shoes are forever conjoined. She mostly wears bedroom ballerina slippers and her 1960s Birkenstocks because she can't find shoes that fit—her foot is too thin, her skin too sensitive, her sole too ouchy. Shoe shopping with her was an exercise in futility.

"I'll take you to Westbrook's," I once said. Mr. Westbrook, the sole owner of a local shoe salon, has been a friend of mine for some twenty years. He knows his shoes, how to fit and sell to his tonier, discerning, and podiatrically challenged customers. He stocks a wide variety of European and American shoes in many weird sizes—including quad A, Betty's size. If he doesn't have the size or color, he'll order it.

Excitedly Betty chose a half dozen pair to try on. Mr. Westbrook measured her foot, disappeared into the back room, and returned, smiling, with nine boxes. He sat on a stool at her feet, in the marriage-proposal position. Holding a shoe up, he looked at her to see if indeed she is Cinderella.

Mr. Westbrook added pads, broke counters, removed pads, softened edges, added arch supports, took away arch supports, offered silk socks, workout socks, no socks.

"No," Betty said after each adjustment. "They don't fit. They hurt *here,*" pointing each time to a different spot. She bought nothing.

I was embarrassed, angry, guilty, and sorry to have brought this client from hell to my friend's store. Betty was disappointed with and angry at me for having raised her hopes.

I realize as I write this that Betty did her shoe shopping the way she's doing her dying: getting lots of help, none of it right, and always pointing to a different spot—back, ribs, feet, lungs, shoulders, head, stomach—that hurts. And me? Still trying to solve problems.

I can empathize with Betty's distress around finding shoes because when I was young and very thin I had trouble finding narrow enough shoes. My ballerina flats were made to order. As a young adult in San Francisco, I lucked onto a shoe shop for models and eventually owned four pairs of fine-fitting shoes.

Two pregnancies, hiking, and jogging have since grown my feet into a nicely average 10B, letting me make up for my earlier shoe deprivation with a shoe wardrobe. I keep each pair of shoes in the original box—complete with packing, tissue, and receipt—on the closet shelf. These mismatched boxes now reach to the ceiling and impinge upon Ernest's shelf space too.

Now I take down each shoe box, open it, and decide whether the shoes are "keepers," "Kidney Foundation," or "trash." A pair of rarely worn Anne Klein strappy black heels that I had bought in NYC with Betty in 1982 I put in the Kidney Foundation pile. A pair of heavy black suede Mephistos bought on the cheap at the Designer Shoe House join the Anne Kleins. Other bargain shoes do too. The newer Ecco, Teva, and Dansko sandals are all keepers. I put the older Tevas in the Kidney Foundation pile. Several pairs of workout shoes go in the trash. Old Eccos join them. I pile the empty mismatched shoe boxes in laundry baskets that are soon overflowing.

From my studio I retrieve two cartons of plastic shoe boxes. I put a pair of keepers in each shoe box and label it by brand and style. Two hours later the boxes are arranged on the shelf by function. I now own "only" twenty-seven pairs.

Am I doing my shoes the way I'll do my dying?

Will I be fortunate enough to have the time and energy to sort through my friends, my groups, my papers, and my activities, holding on to the keepers? Is that not how I want to live my life now? Finding the keepers, letting go of the rest?

"Ernest, will you vacuum the closet floor?" I sweetly ask. Whenever I vacuum, the machine breaks.

Twenty minutes later, Ernest has the closet vacuumed, and I have filled four green garbage bags with cardboard shoe boxes. The tissues I have folded neatly and brought down to my studio.

My body is tired, but my mind is clear.

Thursday, May 18

"Betty," I say on the phone. "Today is the anniversary of that fantastic Horowitz concert. Do you remember it?"

"I think of it often. It was a perfect day."

Friday, May 19

"I have to tell you this," Betty says. She sounds hyper, like she's on "speed." "I've been taking all this prednisone and on Mother's Day 'they' all went to church, which I refused to do because I had nothing to wear. So they sent Mike's mom to come and visit. She stayed for two and a half hours. We have nothing in common but her son. She's so ordinary, it was exhausting, and then Mike's family came. The more people came, the more ashamed I felt—building a four-room apartment and living in only one. I got more and more ashamed and went into a rage. Like a four-year-old. I wanted to break windows and break all the dishes. I wanted to take my car and bulldoze the house. I wanted to take all their cigarettes and smoke them all. This rage went on for hours. It wouldn't go away. . . . Barely dissipated now. . . . Had to do with clothing . . . wanting to get out of the same clothes I've been wearing. . . . I've never experienced anything like this. . . . Felt my brain was totally out of control. . . . Just madness. . . . I'm still mad. . . . Madness."

Saturday, May 20

"Anything good going on?" I ask Betty.

"Sweets! My passion for sweets has returned—chocolate, cake, candy," Betty says. "What about you?"

"My passion for a laptop has returned," I say. "I'm shopping for one to bring with me when I come to Delaware."

"Penny, Jack, Mike, and all of Mike's family will be going to a family reunion first week of July," Betty says. "It would be super if you could come that week. You could stay in Penny's house."

"Not a bad idea," I say. "Let's work on it."

Sunday, May 21

"Do you wish you were back in Kent?" I ask.

Betty mutters.

"I can't hear you," I say. "I can't tell what it is you want, so it is hard for me to support you."

"I don't know what's right. I just don't know."

Thursday, May 25

The memoir writing group meets at Diana's, and I tell them I'm planning on going to Delaware to be the "responsible adult" in Betty's life for the week her family is gone. I'll stay in Penny's house.

"You're a really good friend," Nancy says.

Since October my memoir group has been privy to Betty's ups and downs and my ups and downs.

"When I see her, when I go for my visit, that's when I'll stop writing in this Daybook," I announce. "My visit will mark the end of this book." I imagine an idyllic time like old times—me reading the Daybook out loud, Betty listening, correcting, and laughing. Then she thanks me for writing her stories. And then I imagine she dozes off and I, feeling relieved, do too.

"I'll be able to just enjoy that Betty's still alive," I say, "and I'll be able to get on with my own life. Hal-le-lu-jah!"

Friday, May 26

"Tell me about Ernest's upcoming surgery," Betty asks.

I tell her again that Ernest has two umbilical hernias, and that on June 15 an abdominal surgeon will repair them laparoscopically. Ernest will be forever held together with Dacron mesh, but he'll only be held in Riverside Hospital overnight.

"I have nothing better to do than worry about other people," Betty says. "Everything is closing in on me."

Saturday, May 27

"Hi. I'm walking around," I say to Betty. I am taking my usual neighborhood walk to the end of my street, through Riverlea to the Secret Park, and back again. It's about a mile and a half round trip, and I'm wearing my new and wonderful Tevas. "Whoops! A rock got in my sandal."

"Oh, you mean you're outside," Betty says. "My world is so diminished that I think of 'walking around' as walking around my apartment—in my walker."

Sunday, May 28

My caller ID says "Ellyn G." I pick up immediately.

"Are you okay?" I ask.

"I'm fine," Ellyn says. "Then there's our chronically ill friend. Oy oh oy."

I love hearing Ellyn's New Jersey accent.

"I think Betty would like to be home in Kent, Ohio, and that would be a good place for her now," Ellyn says. "She would have her friends visiting—David, Bonnie, Pam. She wouldn't be so lonely. We have to get her back to Kent for her emotional and psychological health."

"And you're concerned about me going to Delaware while Penny's gone, and being the sole responsible party?" I say.

"Yes, I am." Our shared affection for Betty sustains the strong bond between us. We're commiseration partners. "She'll pull you down. Her need is so huge. She is an empty vessel and no matter what you do you can't fill her up. It's insane for you to go to Delaware. We need to get her back to Kent."

Monday, May 29

At breakfast my sister, Jessica, phones and says, "Are you sure you want to go there, Laurel?"

At lunchtime my friend Julie phones and says, "You may want to rethink your plan."

At dinner Ernest says, "Betty should stay in Delaware. She has a daughter there and the most important thing in her life is her grandson." Family ties trump friendships.

Tuesday, May 30

I tell my Tuesday morning lunch group of my plan to go to Delaware the first week in July and to stay with Betty. Sally looks wary.

"You don't know what you're getting into," Faith says. She's a nurse.

"Wait till next year," Elaine says. She's a nurse too. "Maybe you won't have to go at all."

I laugh. Elaine's a little embarrassed by her dark humor.

"Not a good idea," Cheryl says. She's nurse three. "And *when* is Ernest's double-hernia surgery?"

"June 15. He'll be one night in the hospital."

"And two to six weeks recovering," says Elaine.

Wednesday, May 31

Betty's in the hospital with pleurisy. I look it up on the web. Pleurisy is an inflammation of the lining of the lung, a symptom of an underlying problem. Every breath feels like sandpaper.

"Betty, you can't count on me that first week in July," I tell her. "I'm sorry."

"I know," Betty says.

"I don't know how Ernest's surgery will go."

"Penny shed her first tear today," Betty says. "I was happy to see it."

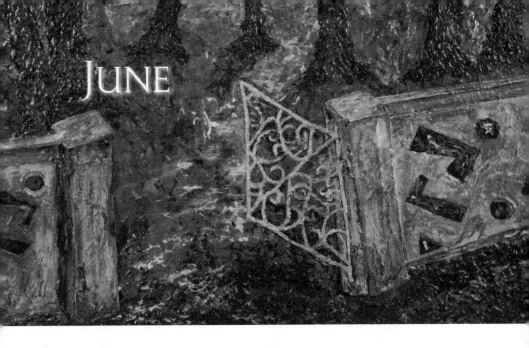

JUNE

Thursday, June 1

"Shopping for Tomorrow." Ernest leaves me a note on the kitchen table telling me where he's gone. He's drawn arrows toward the words and writes, "Good title for your post-Betty book."

Saturday, June 3

"It's funny, but I don't grieve New York City," Betty says. She's in the hospital. "But I always grieve Sedona."

"What do you grieve?" I ask.

"The view. The colors. The sound of Oak Creek."

Sunday, June 4

"I can't read anything. Ten days I've been in this hospital and I haven't read anything. Another loss."

Monday, June 5

"Whatever goes in my obit," Betty says to me on the phone from her hospital bed, "do not say I 'faced illness courageously.' That's so trite. So ordinary."

"Well, Betty," I say, "I won't write that in your obit, but I'll say it to you now. You've been courageous and not at all ordinary. And you still have your dignity." Through all her infirmities, she hasn't complained to the world, only to her dearest friend.

I try to think of something to say that might amuse her, but I can't.

Tuesday, June 6

"Ladies," I say to my Tuesday lunch group. "You'll be happy to know that I am going to Delaware for only three nights, and only if Betty's in assisted living when I visit."

"Good decision," Sally says. "How did Betty take it?"

"It was actually her idea. She's rented us a three-bedroom apartment in Heritage House. I'm up for it. I'll bring her some CDs, look around Dover, maybe go to Rehobeth Beach, maybe go see Penny's house. Betty knows I won't be spending 24/7 with her, about which she is glad. I'd tire her out too much otherwise."

My three nurses nod.

"I'm up for this," I repeat. "It'll give her an opportunity to update her will and obit and tell me what stories she wants in my book." I imagine again that our time together will be like the old times—me stretched on my bed reading her this book, she stretched on hers, pencil and paper in her hands, taking notes, abating my worries, declaring, "It's super, Laurel. Just super. Thanks."

Wednesday, June 7

In addition to the pleurisy, Betty has developed phlebitis. She'll be in the hospital another three days.

"A dear friend of Mike's died, and there is grief everywhere," Betty tells me. "Hundreds of people came to the funeral. That's what happens when you live a long time in the same place. Someone ordered envelopes full of butterflies to be distributed at the funeral. At the right time the envelopes were opened. Everyone's butterfly flew out—everyone's but his wife's. Hers was dead."

I am wincing. "I don't think I could stand that."

My mother died on June 8, 1968. She was sixty-three. A week earlier I had flown to Miami Beach, where my parents had retired—well, Father had, but Mother took on a bookkeeping job because finances were slim. Father didn't believe in taking Social Security.

The first I knew about her cancer was when I helped her into bed and saw her blackened, hardened breast. I don't know how my father could not have known, how he could have ignored it.

"Can't you do something for her?" I yelled at the oncologist. "Surgery or something?"

He looked at me like I was nuts. "Your mother's breast cancer has metastasized. It's in her bones and her brain."

On the morning of June 8, 1968, I felt impelled to drive toward Key West. I called my parents from Long Key. A visiting nurse answered. The doctor had just left. He had given Mother a massive shot of morphine. She had just died. When I got back to Miami Beach, the paramedics were carrying her down the steps in a body bag.

My father wept.

Three years later, homicide police called to tell me that my father was dead. I never saw his body, not even in a body bag.

Today at about 10 p.m. my studio high chair flips over backward with me in it. First my back hits the craft table that has never been screwed into its legs, fortunately. The tabletop flies off, landing on the bookcases, while my body, still encased in the chair, careens onto the oak wood floor. I roll out of the chair, crawl to the hallway, and call up the stairs to Ernest, who can't hear me because he's shaving, getting ready for an early-morning flight to see his grandchildren in San Francisco. I crawl up the stairs and ask Ernest to rub Myoflex on my sore body and to give me a hug. He says, "Be careful."

Friday, June 9

It's nearly 11 p.m. when I notice there is a message on my answering machine.

"Hi," I hear Betty's choked-up voice. I can hear a Schumann piano duet in the background—a CD. Betty must be back in her apartment. "I'm calling for no other reason than that I can pick up the phone and make a phone call. *Cough cough.* At any rate, I hope you're having a good weekend. *Cough cough.* I'll talk to you tomorrow or sometime soon."

I didn't hear the phone ring because at that time I was upstairs in my closet, putting my red Ecco sandals into their new plastic box.

Saturday, June 10

"Hi, Betty," I say. It's 5:00 p.m.

"You always call at the wrong time," she says. Her breathing is very labored, rough.

"I don't *always* call at the wrong time," I say defensively. Then I back off and state the obvious, "You're having trouble breathing."

"I just walked the six steps to the bathroom."

"With your walker?"

"Y—e—ssss."

I hear that rough, crackling noise again.

"I'll call you back," I say.

"I'll call you," Betty says. "In five minutes."

Twenty minutes pass before my phone rings. "As long as I keep the Xanax level I do better," Betty says.

"So what will you do this evening?" I ask.

"Watch reruns of *Law and Order.*"

"Have you thought of audiobooks?"

"I keep falling asleep, and then I have the repetitive dream of someone taking razor blades to my eyes."

"I guess your unconscious has decided against cataract surgery then."

"Why bother making a decision when twenty minutes later I'm open to changing it. So Ernest's gone for a few days. . . . How're you doing?"

"I've had a great day," I say. "I went to the opening of *Speaking Volumes: The Art of the Altered Book.* I have three books in the show!"

"Nancy Drew?" Betty asks.

"No, but a photo of my altered Gail Sheehy book, *New Passages: Mapping Your Life Across Time,* is on the show's poster. The poster calls me 'artist.' On the acknowledgments page, I wrote the names of the women who have been my friends, supporters, and mentors in gold calligraphy. The page was full, top to bottom. Your name is right there on the top!"

"Best friends," she says. I imagine her teary-eyed. I am.

"I'm so inspired that I've come home and begun work on an 'art book.' I'm calling it *Red*."

"You're doing something different in your space alone," she says. "Oh?"

"You're doing what you're doing *happily*."

I let her comment pass, knowing I'll turn it over in my mind later.

"I think *Red* will be about *The Red Shoes*, and the movie's impact on my life," I say.

"That was one of the first movies I ever saw," Betty says.

I want to talk more about *The Red Shoes*, but I can hear how difficult her breathing has become.

"Talk to you later."

"You bet."

Sunday, June 11

I've chosen a blank book with gold-leaf edges, and I've gathered up everything in my studio that is red—cloth, papers, stickers, wrappings, fruit nets, street detritus, cellophane, magazine cutouts—and I have piled them on a work table. I've never worked on an altered book this way before, but as I look at the pile of stuff I have brought to the table, I realize that I am recreating in the material world my way of going about writing. When I write, I know that all my interior "stuff" is there to be sorted out, some chosen, some unexpectedly realigned or reimagined, some discarded. How I write is how I live. How I hope to do my dying.

I rename the book *Meditations on Red*.

Monday, June 12

"I have a question for you," I tell Betty. "Well, two. First, how're you?" She sounds very weak.

"Bad today. I'm in so much pain. My back hurts again. I've had it before."

"From coughing, I think," I say, realizing that her osteoporosis has advanced. Her back bones are fracturing.

"If I can get some Xanax, I'll be okay. But my doctor won't write a mail-in prescription unless I come into his office."

"Can you do that?"

"I'm much too weak."

I wonder if this doctor is afraid that Betty will purposefully OD if he gives her the prescription.

I raise my second question: when to have the nasal turbinate surgery recently ordered by my ENT doctor to help my sleeping. Does she think that July 28 makes sense? Is it long enough after Ernest's hernia surgery, my visit to Delaware, and my birthday, and far enough away from my hoped-for visit to my sister in Des Moines? I don't really need Betty's "advice," but it is a long and good habit, bouncing stuff like this off her, hearing myself think.

"Off to the chiropractor," I say. "Talk to you later."

"You bet."

It's an easy five-minute drive to Gretchen's office. She's on time and adjusts me. As I drive out of her parking lot, a man, whose gray hair peaks out beneath his red dye job, hits the wheel of my Chrysler 300M with his Lexus.

"Maybe I shouldn't be driving anymore," he says. "This is the second time I've hit someone in two days. Maybe I'm too old."

I take his license plate number, and Gretchen readjusts me. Driving toward the Village Bookstore to look for art books, I am feeling completely happy.

I pick up my dear son Josh, who has been offered two auto-service jobs and tells me my front wheel needs to be realigned, and I pick up my grandson, Akiva, who tells me he does not want to go to any camp this summer. I enlist both of them to put my Netflix copy of *The Red Shoes* into the DVD player. Our equipment, Josh quips, is as old as he is.

I saw the premier showing of *The Red Shoes* with my father at the Schubert Theater in downtown Chicago. I was ten. I wore my new wine-colored coat with the real leopard lining over my new red velvet dress.

Other little girls were in red dresses too. My father and I sat in the loge, and, looking down, I thought the girls looked like corsages of red roses. Our fathers in their dark suits were our branches.

Music, dance, color, European cities, English and French accents, and Moira Shearer's sheer beauty entranced my soul. My child mind decided that a woman could have a marriage and a career *only* if she chose a husband who would "let" her. That was my script for choosing my first husband.

About twenty years ago I saw the movie again. That time I saw that a woman could not "have it all"—career, marriage, children—without "killing herself." I thought about how both my parenting and my career had suffered because I had tried to do everything simultaneously, and that nevertheless I could not have done it otherwise. The same, I think, was true for Betty. Not many of us in our generation made that double choice.

When I watch the movie tonight, to my complete surprise, I identify with the ballet impresario, Lermontov. His dream, discipline, and desire to "create . . . to make something big out of something small" touch my heart. When he cries at the end of movie, I do too.

The conflicted ballerina who resonated with my younger self no longer controls my thought, adventures, experiences. I am the impresario of my life.

Tuesday, June 13

"Good morning, Ernest," I say. He arrived home in the wee morning hours from San Francisco. During his layover in Las Vegas he lost forty dollars on the slots and bought me a Las Vegas T-shirt. I call Betty to confirm that once again Ernest's gambling luck is the opposite of hers. Life feels back to normal. My spirits are high. After lunch with my Tuesday lunch group, I drive to Stampland to check out their closing-out sale. I buy a handmade card to send to Betty. On the card a woman hoists a huge watering can, sprinkling an array of flowers. The words say, "If I had a single flower for every time I thought of you, I could walk forever in my garden."

Wednesday, June 14

"How's your back, Betty?" I ask.

"Awful."

"Sorry to hear that," I say. "Things are good here."

"It's freezing here. Like the middle of winter."

"Why is that?" I ask. Something about the importance of winter floats in my brain, but I can't uncover it. A dream I had maybe, . . . but I can't retrieve it.

"There's one air-conditioner for the whole house. I can't control my apartment. Brrr. I'm so cold."

"Can you get another blanket?" I ask. "Or have them turn the air-conditioner down?"

"Always solving problems, aren't you Laurel?"

"You bet," I say, imitating Betty's accent.

"Talk to you later," she says, imitating mine.

Thursday, June 15

"Hi, Betty." I am walking in a corridor in Riverside Hospital, where Ernest has undergone hernia surgery. It's about noon. I am wearing my Las Vegas T-shirt and my strand of pearls, for "good luck and a long life." "He had three hernias," I tell her. "Not one. Not two. Three. Count them: one two three! Just like Ernest to be excessive."

We laugh.

"And how are you?" I ask. "Your back was bothering you yesterday."

"This has been a good day," she says.

"That's good," I say.

"Thanks for calling," she says.

When I replay this conversation in my head, I remember not saying, "Talk to you later," and Betty not saying, "You bet."

"Do you mind if I go to my memoir writing group for a couple hours this afternoon?" I ask Ernest, after seeing him safely ensconced in his hospital bed, tethered to a multitasking IV drip machine. He'll be there two nights.

"Of course not," he says. "Enjoy yourself."

I bring two pieces of writing about Betty to the group. They've come to care about her too.

It is 7:59 p.m. I am talking to my sister, Jessica, when I here the click-click noise that tells me I am getting a voicemail. It's Penny. "Give me a call when you have a chance," she says. She sounds sad, unlike herself. Penny called me when her mother was in intensive care some months ago. I imagine that's what's happening now.

When I return the call, Mike answers the phone. His voice is broken too. "Here. I'll let you talk to Penny."

"Mom passed away tonight," she tells me. "About an hour ago."

"What?" I am in shock. *So this is what shock feels like. Numbness. Surreal. As if I could rewind the clock and make everything okay.* I say, "I talked to her at noon. She said she was having a good day."

"I don't know what happened," Penny says. "The doctor doesn't either. I gave her dinner and went into the yard. She called me on my cell phone, but I couldn't hear her talk. When I came in, she was sitting in her chair. She patted her left lung area and said, 'pain pill, pain pill.' I got her the pill and some tea but she couldn't swallow it. I called EMT. She was unconscious. She was in ER. I followed her living will. She didn't want to be intubated. She was gone. I don't know if it was respiratory failure or a heart attack or a blood clot. The doctor doesn't know either. It wasn't choking on food. She was tired of fighting. It was expected, but not expected."

It seems unreal to me. Five hours ago I was at memoir group reading this sentence: "If Betty is not who she was, who is dying?" Now I know who was dying. I mean who has died. *My best friend has died.* She is not a collection of thoughts and talks and tics and tacks. The whole is much greater than the sum of its parts. Who Betty became this past nine months was more—and less—than who she was.

Me too. I'm more and I'm less.

I am teary, but I don't cry.

I am in shock.

I wish Ernest were home.

"I want to have the memorial service on Tuesday in Kent," Penny continues.

"This Tuesday?" I ask. I can hardly get my mind around it being so soon. "At Bonnie's?"

"Yeah. I want to get this behind me."

I call my sister and tell her the sad news.

I am at loose ends.

This was not how it was supposed to be.

I don't call Ernest at the hospital. Why disturb his sleep?

I clutch my pearls.

I am alone.

I don't know what to do.

I do my e-mail and make popcorn.

My dearest friend has passed away and my plans to finish this book in my own way have been shattered. My plans to visit and to tie up loose ends for her and for me are over. Death trumps life.

Friday, June 16

I wake up thinking, *Something is different today.*

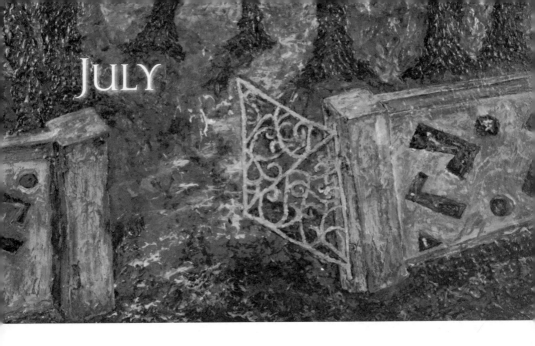

JULY

Saturday, July 15

In my dream, Betty is dressed in white, reclining on a white chaise. Her skin is smooth and peach-toned, her hair soft and curled, her body fuller. She looks like a Degas. I am wearing pearls, standing facing her, showing her a travel map of California. It's printed on one 8½-by-11-inch sheet of writing paper.

I say, "I guess we won't be driving down the coast road together, down Route 1."

Betty says, "Don't be so sure of that, Laurel."

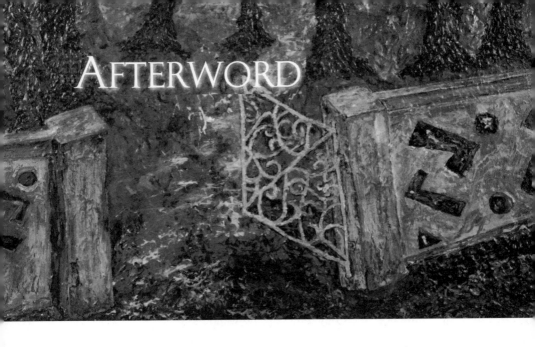

AFTERWORD

On January 15, 2007, I mailed a copy of *Last Writes: A Daybook for a Dying Friend* to the Left Coast Press, Inc., situated some forty miles inland from California's coastal Route 1. It felt terrific sending the manuscript there. Perhaps the dream I had on July 15, 2006, was prophetic, for with the Left Coast Press, Inc. as publisher, my best friend, Betty, and I are indeed taking a trip together down California's Route 1.

Best friends is not just a label hyped by nine-year-olds. It's a wondrous truth in the lives of many grown-ups. Betty and I were best friends for thirty-five years. Like other best friends, we saw each other through many of life's passages, joys, and sorrows, and we turned to each other for support, caring, help—and fun.

When her physician told me that Betty's pulmonary disease had reached the stage where she had at best a few months to live, my first thought was, *I don't know how I'll live my life without her.* I turned to my Daybook where, habitually, near daily, I write about my stress, fears, and anxieties, shaping them and coming to understand them through writing. I wrote about the progress of her illness, our complex and sometimes difficult friendship, and my conflicting emotions: grief, despair, anger, disgust, love. And I wrote about what I was doing with my life—traveling, visiting friends, writing—while she was in the midst of a painful dying.

My memory for events, places, and spoken words was trained since I was a preschooler (see April 1), and has been developed in my career as a qualitative researcher and interviewer. I am comfortable describing settings, keeping notes, writing up conversations, as well as inventorying and expressing my feelings through writing (see October 9).

Writing in the Daybook helped me get through the final nine months of Betty's life. Writing kept me alive to the immanence of illness in her life—and its shadow on mine. Keeping the Daybook was therapeutic. It gave me a space to vent my emotions, record her end-of-life stories, our shared experiences, and chronicle the "good days and bad days" phenomenon of chronic illness—and wellness.

The Daybook format allowed the inclusion of dreams, poetry, e-mails, and letters, and allowed exploration of my feelings through recreating scenes and reporting remembered conversations. I was free to write whatever I wanted to write and to write it however I chose to write it.

I realized that what I was experiencing was not extraordinary. The death of friends is an increasingly prevalent fact for baby boomers, as is the dependence of women upon each other during illnesses. I thought my Daybook could illuminate "ordinary" women's lives—and deaths.

I decided that I wanted *Last Writes: A Daybook for a Dying Friend* to be published. But writing for an audience is different from writing for the self. The former has many external constraints, the later has none. So I knew I would have to address several writing and ethical issues before the book could leave its cloistered life.

When publishing about other people, my ethics require that I subject my writing to a fine-mesh filter: do no harm. What should I reveal? To whom should it be revealed, when, and how?

Of course, no matter what precautions we take, no matter how painstakingly we filter what we say and how we say it, we cannot know the consequences of our work. We can only do the best we can. One way to help us do the best we can is to give the people we write about a chance to preview what we have written—but not necessarily the right to alter or delete the text (what others have called "member check"). Keeping the control of the text with its author, I think, is especially important when one is writing personal narrative such as memoir or daybook. It is the author's story, after all.

There are many people besides me in *Last Writes*: my husband, my family, friends, colleagues, administrators, royalty, strangers, and, of course, my best friend, Betty, plus her family, friends, and physicians. I used different strategies for sharing the prepublished manuscript with different people. I'll talk about the writing decisions concerning the people less central to the narrative first, turning to a discussion of Betty later.

My husband, Ernest Lockridge, appears throughout the Daybook, but it was not until I began writing this afterword that I realized I never asked him for permission to talk about him or quote him. Why is that? The most obvious answer is that we enjoy a level of intimacy and trust that will not be violated in my writing. The less obvious answer is that I read this book to him while I was writing it. He had the tacit opportunity, should he have chosen to take it, to request changes in the manuscript. Once he did. I had left out an important conversation with him that he thought belonged in the manuscript—not because of his ego but because it contributed to the narrative's strength (see October 11). But he never asked me to delete my droll asides (for example, see April 14). Ethically, though, I would have deleted them had he found them painful rather than funny. They add little to the arc of the narrative, but they do tell the reader about our relationship and my penchant for droll humor.

My siblings, children, and grandchildren appear sporadically, and for the most part positively. But I have revealed some of my younger son's challenges. I asked him to vet my writing about him, which he declined. "I trust you, Mom," he said. "Anyone can know anything about me." This carte blanche is both heartening and frightening to me, for perhaps some of the things "anyone might know about him" might reflect poorly on me and his family. But that's life. There is no way to be shielded from potshots or negative evaluations. But there is a way to limit the pain they might produce, and that is by taking charge of the narrative myself, telling my own story. It is better, I have found, to be the revealer rather than the revealed. The February 4 entry is an example of this.

Many of my friends, individually and as group members, appear in the book. All of them read their "parts" in the narrative and gave permission to use their names and to quote them. I thought of sharing the manuscript as a courtesy, a useful fact-checking technique, and incidentally a way to receive feedback on my writing. All but one of my friends were pleased to be in my book and asked that I use their real names.

The one friend who took exception said she was surprised that I had taken what she had thought of as a private conversation and put it in my book. I was surprised at her surprise. She is cast in a wholly positive light, and I note her eloquent observations. She is a fellow academic who I had thought was familiar with my published personal narratives. She gave me permission to use the conversation "if it fit into the book," but I could hear her hesitancy. I decided to change her name and all identifying characteristics. Does she feel I misused our friendship, capitalized on it for my writing ventures? I sense unease between us. Have I alienated a dear friend of twenty-five years? Could I have done it differently? Should I do it differently? Doing what I thought of as a courtesy call has challenged my friend's trust in me. I cannot repair that breach, but I can work to prevent its widening, which I have done by asking her about it now. "You're more sensitive to the issues than I am," she said. "I'm fine." Yet there still lingers in me the need to continue doing the emotional repair work.

On the other hand, to my surprise my contact in Australia chose not to read the manuscript before it was published. I puzzled over why. The answer is actually rather simple. If I treat her supervisors (or colleagues) poorly—and she has reason to suspect that I might do so—and if she has read the manuscript and not insisted that I change it, she could be viewed as complicit and might be punished by her supervisors. Sometimes, then, the best ethical choice is to not share the text prepublication.

My Australian contact (whose name and identifiers I have changed) was actually wise, I think, in choosing not to read the manuscript for, although I thoroughly disguise one of her supervisors and several members of the Australian royalty, I treat them with a bit of dry humor (see March 9). Why do I think drollery is ethical? I routinely make fun of myself too when I'm acting "too big for my britches," and of my husband when he's too big for his, and of anyone whom I experience as putting on airs, including the hapless bookstore owner who ignores me (see March 3 to 5). Dry humor is a writing technique, a tone choice that humanizes rather than demonizes, showing the reader that I value down-to-earthness. If, in a personal narrative, I were to write against that value, I would be acting dishonestly.

Of all the people in the book, the one I was most concerned about hurting was Betty's daughter, Penny. At the end of her life, a cantankerous Betty was living with her daughter miles from her home and friends in Kent. Betty criticized her daughter's way of life—a down-to-earth, rural one—that I make clear in the book I admire (see March 15). Although I thought it unlikely that Penny would know about this book, I would feel I had betrayed her if I published it before she had a chance to read it. I asked her if she wanted to use her real name. She did. After considerable thought, however, I decided to override her request. I changed all identifiers because I could not gauge how her in-laws might respond and because her eight-year-old son is too young to give informed consent.

When Penny's e-mail arrived thanking me for the manuscript and saying she "loved it," I was greatly relieved. Her response to her mother's criticism of Penny's way of life—the critical part of the book I most worried about—is worth quoting: "I never thought of our life as ordinary or boring but I guess it is. I kind of like this small town existence—it's funny because there is a whole shift back to this 'slower' way. Burning the candle at both ends is not a problem here because people don't let it become an issue. Too many garages to visit." Penny's reading of Betty's negative opinion, rather than being distressing, increased Penny's sense of value in the life she had chosen for herself. How often, I wonder, do we as writers of other people's lives expend our energies "protecting" our subjects from our words, when those words might be a source of regeneration for them?

Writing about the death of a best friend has presented challenging writing issues. Betty grew up as an East Coast secular Jew with three commandments: plant a tree, raise a child, write a book. The first two she accomplished on her own; the third has rested with me. Betty desired that I "tell her stories" and give her the "immortality" that she believed only published writing could give (see February 28; May 9). How was I to do this? My ideas about what was "right" to write and how to write evolved through the writing, and through her dying. Writing choices and ethics merged.

For the first few months of Betty's dying process, I wrote to record her experiences and my feelings. I worked on developing my skills at writing dialogue and scenes, not because of publication issues but because my Daybook was a *writer's daybook,* a place for me to hone my craft while exploring my fears and angers. I must have known, in my subconscious, however, that something more was going on because I became aware of my moving into interviewer mode, asking questions and recording answers as if I were collecting data for some future project (see October 26).

But in February, when I realized I was writing a book for publication, ethical questions bombarded me. I chose not to tell Betty about the book because I was unsure if it would hurt her or inhibit her. Would she distort, lie, or conceal her end-of-life experiences if she knew I was writing about her, and if she knew would it inevitably alter our friendship? I was the sole repository of her stories, complaints, and issues. I was her best friend. The project of writing the book might have superseded the project of dying.

I did not have the imagination to suggest both/and—that is, telling her about the book and initiating off-the-record conversations. In retrospect, I think this was good, given my experience using another friend's conversation and losing her trust. But what happened instead was the gradual confirmation that she indeed wanted me to write this book. "Tell my stories," she said. "Let them know I did more with my life than my measly obituary." So writing her stories, I have felt, has had her blessing. And for the most part, I have chosen to tell her stories as she presented them to me, through dialogue and scenes.

One of the larger stories of her life, though, the May 4 shootings at Kent State University, I chose to tell through my own voice. I needed to write an account in which no blame was laid. My own ethics of "reporting" a historical event took precedence over ethical considerations of reporting Betty's take on it. Although I had a pretty good sense of what she thought, she was already too ill to talk about it. Writing from the vantage of her Kent State friends, who probably shared her viewpoint, would move too far from the book's narrative arc, I felt. Writing May 4 as I did I reconfirmed that this was *my* narrative—mine to shape (see May 7).

I conjectured about her thoughts and actions, some of which I did not admire. Nevertheless, I decided to keep them in the book for both writerly and ethical reasons. Any long-term friendship, such as our thirty-five-year one, is going to be riddled with angers, resentments, missteps, and renewals. Any long-term friendship is going to be challenged by the changes that will inevitably happen to each friend. People can grow apart; friends can negotiate a way back. My Daybook, I realized, was presenting an exemplar of a difficult friendship and how friends could transcend their differences.

So I have done more in this book than tell Betty's stories. I have told mine too. We began our friendship similar to each other in many ways, and I used that similarity to ground the book in the literary device of doubling—from the concrete double strand of pearls and duplicate bridge to repetitious playful language, such as "lugging luggage," "Ernest earnestly," and "Shearer's sheer beauty." The reader will find many other examples. This is a technique that grew from the unconscious and deep truth about our relationship. As our later lives unfold, I am traveling about the world as she lies dying. Betty becomes her "own shadow," and "my shadow, double, sister."

Writing about Betty's death and dying has had a transformative effect on me. I am clearer about my priorities, happier in my choices, and less certain about how I'll go through my own death and dying—less smug and superior. In deep pain toward the end, Betty was cantankerous and curmudgeonly, but never downright mean, ugly, or fearful. She never let go of the desire to be alive in this world.

She kept her dignity and sense of humor. I hope I will be able to do the same.

I had planned to see Betty in mid-June and read her this Daybook. I had planned to enjoy the rest of her life *as a life*, and not as a subject. In graduate school I had a sign on my desk: Life is what happens when you're making plans. Now I know that death is what happens too.